CONTENTS

W9-AAO-287

Good Living With Fibromyalgia
WORKBOOK

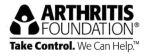

An Official Publication
of the Arthritis Foundation

Published by
Arthritis Foundation
1330 West Peachtree Street
Atlanta, GA 30309

Printed in Canada
2nd Printing 2003

Library of Congress Card Catalog Number: 2002100857

ISBN: 0-912-423-35-8

Order ID: 104-8649084-2453057

Thank you for buying from Anaheim UMC on Amazon Marketplace.

Shipping Address:		Order Date:	Nov 20,
Suzanne Wright		Shipping Service:	Standard
55 McKinstry Ave		Buyer Name:	Suzanne
Peru, IN 46970-2804		Seller Name:	Anaheim

Quantity	Product Details
1	**The Good Living With Fibromyalgia Workbook: Activites for a Better Life (Gu** **Merchant SKU:** LY-LHD5-XQEZ **ASIN:** 0912423358 **Listing ID:** 1103I8VAFE5 **Order-Item ID:** 21994851634466 **Condition:** Used - Like New

Returning your item:
Go to "Your Account" on Amazon.com, click "Your Orders" and then click the "seller profile" link for th
information about the return and refund policies that apply.
Visit http://www.amazon.com/returns to print a return shipping label. Please have your order ID ready.

Thanks for buying on Amazon Marketplace. To provide feedback for the seller please visit
www.amazon.com/feedback. To contact the seller, please visit Amazon.com and click on "Your Account
any page. In Your Account, go to the "Orders" section and click on the link "Leave seller feedback". Sele
click on the "View Order" button. Click on the "seller profile" under the appropriate product. On the lower
the page under "Seller Help", click on "Contact this seller".

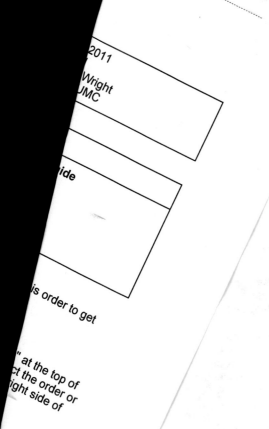

2011

Wright
UMC

ide

is order to get

" at the top of
ct the order or
ight side of

ACKNOWLEDGEMENTS

The *Good Living with Fibromyalgia Workbook* is written for people with fibromyalgia who want to take charge of their condition and their lives. This book is a companion guide to *The Arthritis Foundation's Guide to Good Living with Fibromyalgia*, also published by the Arthritis Foundation.

This book was reviewed by John H. Klippel, MD, President and CEO of the Arthritis Foundation; Laurence Bradley, PhD, of the University of Alabama, Birmingham; Patricia Grosklaus, PT, of Atlanta, GA; Kathleen S. Lewis, RN, author of *Celebrate Life,* of Decatur, GA; and Marjory Vals Maud of Chandler, AZ, an Arthritis Foundation volunteer and certified leader of the Arthritis Foundation's Fibromyalgia Self-Help Course.

Portions of this book were inspired by the Arthritis Foundation's Fibromyalgia Self-Help Course, a program of self-management developed in the late 1980s and originally supported by the Norma Borie Fibromyalgia Research and Education Program Fund, and by the Chronic Disease Self-Management Course, developed by Kate Lorig, RN, DrPH, and her colleagues at the Stanford Arthritis Center. The Arthritis Foundation wishes to thank Dr. Lorig and her colleagues for their efforts on behalf of educating people with fibromyalgia.

Special thanks go to Bethany Afshar, who wrote the text. The editorial director of the book is Susan Bernstein. The art director of the book and the designer of the cover is Susan Siracusa. Layout was completed by Jill Dible.

INTRODUCTION

You are in the driver's seat when it comes to managing your fibromyalgia. There are many turns along the road to good living, and you need the right map to help you make the best decisions. This book, *The Good Living With Fibromyalgia Workbook,* is designed to help you find the way to a better, healthier, more fulfilling life with fibromyalgia.

Don't just read this workbook from beginning to end and then put it down. Instead, read the chapters and complete the activities as they apply to you on a daily basis. Use this workbook as a daily companion to help you manage your fibromyalgia more successfully.

Despite the pain, anxiety, fatigue and other symptoms you may be experiencing, this book has activities and interactive features that will help you discover the techniques and options that will help you achieve that goal of good living with fibromyalgia. You'll learn how to identify your symptoms and their possible causes. You'll learn about the many drugs and other therapies used to treat your pain, fatigue or other problems. Most of all, you'll learn techniques that will put you in control of your fibromyalgia – not the other way around.

It's important that you work with your doctor and other health-care professionals – your "health-care team" – to create effective strategies for dealing with your fibromyalgia. But, after all, the most important member of your health-care team is *you.* With this workbook, you'll learn how to achieve good living with fibromyalgia.

If you seek more in-depth information about your fibromyalgia, this workbook is a companion to the book *The Arthritis Foundation's Guide to Good Living With Fibromyalgia.* Call 800/207-8633 or log on to www.arthritis.org for more information about this valuable resource on fibromyalgia.

The mission of the Arthritis Foundation is to improve lives through leadership in the prevention, control and cure of arthritis and related diseases.

GOOD LIVING
GOOD LIVING
GOOD LIVING
GOOD LIVING
GOOD LIVING
GOOD LIVING
GOOD LIVING
GOOD LIVING
GOOD LIVING

CHAPTER 1:

Understanding Fibromyalgia

Understanding how and why you hurt may be the first step in managing your fibromyalgia. You may be experiencing sharp pains or an all-over sort of ache. You may have difficulty sleeping or feel exhausted all day long.

Fibromyalgia is a mysterious condition that is baffling to people who have it and the doctors who treat it. There is no known cure for fibromyalgia, and researchers continue to investigate its cause. To ensure that you are receiving the best care and doing all you can for your fibromyalgia, you need to understand fibromyalgia and what it is doing to your body.

What Is Fibromyalgia?

Fibromyalgia is an arthritis-related condition that is characterized by generalized pain and fatigue. The term *fibromyalgia* means pain in the muscles, ligaments and tendons. The condition also is characterized by its common symptoms. See page 4 for a complete list of symptoms.

Fibromyalgia is a confusing and often misunderstood condition. Because its symptoms are quite common and laboratory tests are generally normal, fibromyalgia patients once were told that their condition was "all in their head." However, medical studies have proven that fibromyalgia does indeed exist, and it is estimated to affect about 3.7 million Americans today.

It wasn't until 1990 that fibromyalgia was legitimized in the medical community. That year, the American College of Rheuma-tology (ACR), the official body of doctors who specialize in arthritis and related diseases, presented its criteria for diagnosing fibro-myalgia. It is diagnosed when the patient has the following symptoms:

- A history of widespread pain (pain on both sides of the body and above and below the waist) that is present for at least three months;

- Pain in at least 11 of 18 tender-point sites (see opposite page).

The Diagnosis Dilemma

The difficulty with diagnosing someone with fibromyalgia is that there is no clear-cut test to determine fibromyalgia. No evidence of it appears on X-rays or in laboratory test results. There is no diagnostic marker in the blood. People with fibromyalgia often look healthy, with no outward signs of pain or fatigue.

Instead, fibromyalgia is diagnosed by the identification of symptoms – widespread pain plus tender points – and the exclusion of other conditions. Doctors use laboratory

tests to rule out other conditions with similar symptoms, such as thyroid conditions.

The diagnostic process can take years, partly due to the fact that fibromyalgia remains unfamiliar to many people, including doctors. Fortunately, a greater understanding of fibromyalgia now exists within the medical community. Finding the right doctor can help expedite diagnosis. For tips on choosing a doctor, see "Choose Your Doctor Wisely," page 36.

ACTIVITY

Tender Points

Tender points are areas of the body that are sensitive to pressure. Although fibromyalgia is diagnosed by finding pain in these specific tender points, people with fibromyalgia may experience pain and tenderness virtually all over the body.

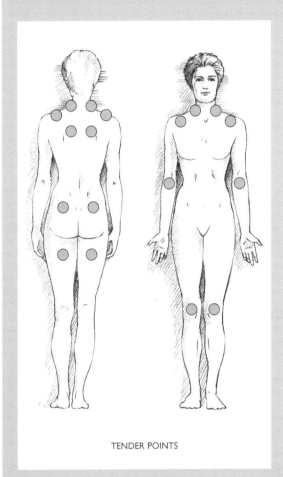

TENDER POINTS

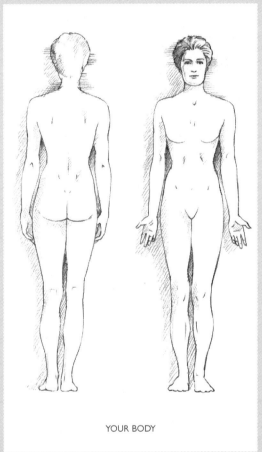

YOUR BODY

WHERE DO YOU HURT?

The 18 tender points doctors examine to help determine a diagnosis of fibromyalgia are shown on the above left image. Using the image on the right, mark your tender points and where you hurt the most.

Common Symptoms

Although no two people with fibromyalgia experience the same symptoms the exact same way, people with fibromyalgia do experience similar symptoms. Here are the most common fibromyalgia symptoms:

PAIN

By far the most prominent of fibromyalgia symptoms, pain – either regionally or all-over – differs from person to person. Some people with fibromyalgia describe their pain as knife-like in intensity, while others compare it to an all-over muscle cramp.

FATIGUE

Up to 80 percent of people with fibromyalgia experience fatigue. Fatigue may include feelings of listlessness, decreased exercise endurance, mental or physical exhaustion or sleepiness that varies from day to day and throughout the day.

SLEEP DISTURBANCE

As many as 90 percent of people with fibromyalgia have abnormal sleep patterns. They often have difficulty falling asleep or staying asleep, or they sleep extremely lightly.

DEPRESSION AND ANXIETY

Although they don't go hand-in-hand, depression is common in many people with fibromyalgia. People with fibromyalgia often report feeling "blue" or "down," although only approximately 25 percent are considered clinically depressed, a condition requiring the care of a mental-health professional.

COGNITIVE DIFFICULTIES

Many people with fibromyalgia experience cognitive disturbances, otherwise known as *fibro fog*, which can be characterized by feelings of confusion, lapses in memory, word mix-ups and difficulty concentrating.

OTHER SIGNS AND SYMPTOMS

Many other physical problems may accompany fibromyalgia, causing additional pain, discomfort and frustration. They include:

- Headaches – muscular, tension or migraine
- Irritable bowel syndrome – a condition marked by alternating constipation and diarrhea
- Skin color changes – a temporary change because of sensitivity to temperature and moisture
- Tingling limbs – hands, arms, feet, legs or face feel numb or as if they've "fallen asleep"
- Jaw pain – such as temporomandibular joint (TMJ) disorder
- Restless legs syndrome – a condition that causes the legs to jump or spasm during sleep

For more information about the symptoms of fibromyalgia, see Chapter 1 of *The Arthritis Foundation's Guide to Good Living With Fibromyalgia*. (Call 800/207-8633 or visit www.arthritis.org to order.)

What Are Your Symptoms?

Because fibromyalgia is a condition made up of many different symptoms, it is important for you to know which symptoms you have and which are most troubling for you. Check the boxes below next to the symptoms you have, and share this information with your doctor.

❏ **PAIN** – Is it all-over or regional? Is it a sharp, stabbing feeling or general achiness? Please describe: _____

_____

(For pain-management tips, see page 122.)

❏ **FATIGUE** – Do you tire quickly? Do you just feel spent? Do you feel tired during the day? Please describe: _____

_____

(For ways to battle fatigue, see page 134.)

❏ **SLEEP DISTURBANCE** – Do you have trouble falling asleep or staying asleep? Do you feel tired even after sleeping through the night? Please describe:_____

_____

(For pointers for a better night's sleep, see page 143.)

❏ **DEPRESSION/ANXIETY** – Are you often "down" or "blue"? Are you prone to feeling anxious? Please describe:_____

_____

(To test yourself for depression, see page 161.)

❏ **COGNITIVE DIFFICULTIES (FIBRO FOG)** – Are you constantly forgetting where you put your keys, glasses, etc.? Do you mix up words or lose your train of thought in mid-sentence? Please describe: _____

_____

(For tips on dealing with fibro fog, see page 18.)

❏ **IRRITABLE BOWEL SYNDROME (IBS)** – Do you have constipation, diarrhea, abdominal cramps, bloating, gas or other digestive difficulties? Please describe: _____

_____

(To see what you can do about IBS, see page 21.)

continued page 6

What Are Your Symptoms? continued

❏ **HEADACHES** – Are your headaches stress- or diet-related? Do you suffer from migraines? Please describe: _____

_____

_____

(To learn more about common headache triggers, see page 20.)

❏ **SKIN SENSITIVITY** – Is your skin extremely sensitive to touch or to temperature changes? Please describe: _____

_____

_____

❏ **TINGLING LIMBS** – Do your hands or feet go numb or have a "pins and needles" sensation? Are your arms or legs falling asleep a lot? Please describe: _____

_____

_____

❏ **PAINFUL JAW** – Does your jaw hurt sometimes? Have you been diagnosed with temporomandibular joint (TMJ) disorder? Please describe: _____

_____

_____

❏ **RESTLESS LEGS SYNDROME (RLS)** – Do your legs seem to have a mind of their own sometimes? Do they twitch when you sleep? Please describe: _____

_____

_____

(For more information about RLS, see page 144.)

❏ **OTHER** – Please describe: _____

_____

_____

_____

_____

_____

_____

_____

_____

GOOD LIVING
GOOD LIVING
GOOD LIVING
GOOD LIVING
GOOD LIVING
GOOD LIVING
GOOD LIVING
GOOD LIVING
GOOD LIVING

GOOD LIVING
GOOD LIVING
GOOD LIVING
GOOD LIVING
GOOD LIVING
GOOD LIVING
GOOD LIVING
GOOD LIVING
GOOD LIVING

CHAPTER 2:

Relieving Symptoms

Fibromyalgia is defined by its symptoms, and treating the condition means managing those symptoms. For you, that may mean quite a mix of therapies, from medications that treat your pain and help you sleep to exercise and relaxation techniques that strengthen your muscles and help reduce stress. Your health-care team will help you find the best balance of treatments to help you live well with fibromyalgia.

Treatment Options

Although there is no known cure for fibromyalgia, its symptoms can be treated using a variety of approaches. A combination of medications and self-management techniques is the key to good living with fibromyalgia. You may benefit from using one or more of the following treatments:

- Moderate exercise, to stretch muscles and improve cardiovascular fitness
- Relaxation techniques, to reduce stress

- Education, to help you understand and cope with the condition
- Healthy habits, such as eating well and not smoking
- Medications, to diminish pain and improve sleep
- Alternative therapies such as acupuncture, massage, or herbs and supplements

Your doctor can help you determine which treatments work best for you.

Medical Therapies

No magic pill exists to treat fibromyalgia. Instead, people with the condition take medications to treat specific symptoms. Your doctor will work with you to determine which medications will work best. This is a trial-and-error process that may take months. Here is a breakdown of medications doctors prescribe for patients with fibromyalgia:

- Tricyclic Antidepressants. Although more commonly used for treating depression, tricyclic antidepressants also relax muscles and restore sleep.
- Selective Serotonin Reuptake Inhibitors (SSRIs). These drugs aid the release of *serotonin* (a hormone that regulates pain and deep sleep) to reduce fatigue, mental confusion, depression and pain.
- Nonsteroidal Anti-Inflammatory Drugs (NSAIDs). Moderate doses of NSAIDs, which include common drugs such as

aspirin and ibuprofen, may relieve pain and stiffness.
- Analgesics. This category of pain relievers encompasses both over-the-counter and prescription medications, including narcotics, which are potent – and potentially addictive – drugs that interrupt pain signals traveling to the brain.
- Benzodiazepines. These tranquilizers can help reduce muscle tension and improve sleep.
- Tender-Point Injections. Injecting a local anesthetic directly into a patient's tender points can provide relief that lasts from hours to several months. These injections are used only in the most severe cases.
- Topical Ointments. Applied directly to the skin on the areas where pain occurs, topical ointments may increase blood flow to the skin, soothing painful muscles, or decrease nerve pain.

Drugs Used in Treating Fibromyalgia

At this time, there are no drugs specifically approved by the Food and Drug Administration for treating fibromyalgia. Here are some drugs that may alleviate certain symptoms associated with fibromyalgia, including pain, sleep problems and muscle aches.

ANALGESICS

These are drugs used for pain relief. Other than acetaminophen, these have the potential for dependence if used for long periods of time.

Acetaminophen
Brand names: *Anacin (aspirin-free), Excedrin caplets, Panadol, Tylenol*
Dosage: 325 to 1,000 mg every 4 to 6 hours as needed, no more than 3,000 mg per day
Possible side effects: When taken as prescribed, acetaminophen usually is not associated with side effects.

Acetaminophen with codeine
Brand names: *Fioricet, Phenaphen with codeine, Tylenol with codeine*
Dosage: 15 to 60 mg every 4 hours as needed
Possible side effects: Constipation, dizziness or lightheadedness, drowsiness, nausea, unusual tiredness or weakness, vomiting

Hydrocodone with acetaminophen
Brand names: *Dolacet, Hydrocet, Lorcet, Lortab, Vicodin*
Dosage: 2.5 to 10 mg every 4 to 6 hours as needed
Possible side effects: Dizziness, drowsiness, lightheadedness or feeling faint, nausea or vomiting, unusual tiredness or weakness

Oxycodone
Brand names: *OxyContin, Roxicodone*
Dosage: For *OxyContin*, 10 mg every 12 hours as needed; for *Roxicodone*, 5 mg every 3 to 6 hours or 10 mg 3 or 4 times a day as needed
Possible side effects: Dizziness, drowsiness, lightheadedness or feeling faint, nausea or vomiting, unusual tiredness or weakness

Propoxyphene hydrochloride
Brand names: *Darvon, PC-Cap, Wygesic*
Dosage: 65 mg every 4 hours as needed, no more than 390 mg per day
Possible side effects: Dizziness or lightheadedness, drowsiness, nausea and vomiting

Tramadol
Brand name: *Ultram*
Dosage: 50 to 100 mg every 6 hours as needed
Possible side effects: Dizziness, nausea, constipation, headache, sleepiness

Drugs Used in Treating Fibromyalgia (continued)

ANTIDEPRESSANTS

Antidepressants, including tricyclics and selective serotonin reuptake inhibitors (SSRIs), help people with fibromyalgia get the deep, restorative sleep they often lack. These drugs are taken in smaller doses than they are when used to treat depression.

TRICYCLICS:

Amitriptyline hydrochloride
Brand name: *Elavil, Endep*
Dosage: 10 to 50 mg per day in a single dose
Possible side effects: Difficulty concentrating, dizziness, drowsiness, dry mouth, headache, increased appetite (including craving for sweets), nausea, sleep disturbances, unpleasant taste, urinary retention, weakness or tiredness, weight gain

Doxepin
Brand name: *Adapin, Sinequan*
Dosage: 10 to 50 mg per day a few hours before bedtime in a single dose
Possible side effects: Difficulty concentrating, dizziness, drowsiness, dry mouth, headache, increased appetite (including craving for sweets), nausea, sleep disturbances, unpleasant taste, urinary retention, weakness or tiredness, weight gain

Nortriptyline
Brand name: *Aventyl, Pamelor*
Dosage: 10 to 50 mg per day a few hours before bedtime in a single dose
Possible side effects: Difficulty concentrating, dizziness, drowsiness, dry mouth, headache, increased appetite (including craving for sweets), nausea, sleep disturbances, unpleasant taste, urinary retention, weakness or tiredness, weight gain

SELECTIVE SEROTONIN REUPTAKE INHIBITORS (SSRIs)

Fluoxetine
Brand name: *Prozac*
Dosage: 10 to 80 mg per day in a single dose
Possible side effects: Anxiety and nervousness, diarrhea, dry mouth, headache, increased sweating, nausea, trouble sleeping

Paroxetine
Brand name: *Paxil*
Dosage: 10 to 40 mg per day in a single dose
Possible side effects: Constipation, decreased sexual ability, dizziness, dry mouth, headache, nausea, difficulty urinating, tremors, trouble sleeping, unusual tiredness or weakness, vomiting

Sertraline
Brand name: *Zoloft*
Dosage: 25 to 100 mg per day in a single dose
Possible side effects: Decreased appetite or weight loss; decreased sexual drive or ability; diarrhea; drowsiness; dryness of the mouth; headache, stomach or abdominal cramps, gas or pain; tremors; trouble sleeping; clumsiness or unsteadiness; dizziness or lightheadedness; drowsiness; slurred speech

BENZODIAZEPINES – SLEEP MEDICATION

Temazepam
Brand name: *Restoril*
Dosage: 15 mg per day in a single dose
Possible side effects: When taken as prescribed, temazepam is not usually associated with side effects.

MUSCLE RELAXANTS

Cyclobenzaprine
Brand names: *Cycloflex, Flexeril*
Dosage: 10 to 40 mg per day best tolerated as a single dose several hours before bedtime
Possible side effects: Dizziness or lightheadedness, drowsiness, dry mouth, confusion

NSAIDS: NONSTEROIDAL ANTI-INFLAMMATORY DRUGS

NSAIDs reduce inflammation, which is not a feature of fibromyalgia, but some people with fibromyalgia may take over-the-counter NSAIDs for mild pain relief. Prescription NSAIDs are available. Talk to your doctor to find out if they can help you.

Note: NSAIDs should be taken with food. Possible side effects for all NSAIDs, except where noted, include abdominal pain, fluid retention, gastric ulcers and bleeding, greater susceptibility to bruising or bleeding from cuts, heartburn, indigestion, lightheadedness, nausea, reduction in kidney function, increase in liver enzymes. COX-2 inhibitors, a new class of NSAID, are less likely to cause gastrointestinal distress or stomach ulcers. If you consume more than three alcoholic drinks per day, check with your doctor before using these products.

Aspirin
Brand names: *Anacin, Ascriptin, Bayer, Bufferin, Ecotrin, Excedrin Tablets, ZORprin, others*
Dosage: 3,600 to 5,400 mg per day in several doses

Drugs Used in Treating Fibromyalgia (continued)

Ibuprofen
Brand names: *Advil, Motrin, Motrin IB, Mediprin, Nuprin*
Dosage: 200 to 400 mg every 4 to 6 hours as needed, not exceeding 1,200 mg per day

Ketoprofen
Brand names: *Actron, Orudis KT*
Dosage: 12.5 mg every 4 to 6 hours as needed

Naproxen sodium
Brand names: *Aleve*
Dosage: 220 mg every 8 to 12 hours as needed

COX-2 INHIBITORS – PRESCRIPTION ONLY

Celecoxib
Brand names: *Celebrex*
Dosage: 200 mg per day in 1 or 2 doses

Rofecoxib
Brand names: *Vioxx*
Dosage: 12.5 mg or 25 mg per day in a single dose

Valdecoxib
Brand names: *Bextra*
Dosage: 10 mg once daily

OTHER DRUGS USED FOR FIBROMYALGIA

Maprotiline
Brand names: *Ludiomil* (another form of antidepressant)
Dosage: 25 to 150 mg per day in 1 to 3 doses
Possible side effects: Blurred vision, decreased sexual ability, dizziness or lightheadedness, drowsiness, dry mouth, headaches, increased or decreased sexual drive, tiredness or weakness

Trazodone
Brand names: *Desyrel, Trazon, Trialodine* (another form of antidepressant)
Dosage: 50 to 150 mg per day in 2 or 3 doses
Possible side effects: Dizziness or lightheadedness, drowsiness, dry mouth, headache, nausea and vomiting, unpleasant taste in mouth

Zolpidem
Brand names: *Ambien* (another form of sleep aid)
Dosage: 10 mg per day in a single dose
Possible side effects: Side effects are uncommon at prescribed dosage.

Talking Drugs With Your Doc

Treating fibromyalgia is a two-way street. You need your doctor to prescribe treatments, offer resources and refer you to other health professionals if needed. Your doctor needs to know that you understand your treatment, how it makes you feel and if you are experiencing any side effects.

Use the following tips to improve communication between you and your doctor:

DO ASK

- What are the possible side effects of the drugs?

- How long should I be prepared to wait for the drug to work?

- What should I do if I miss a dose?

- Are there special instructions for taking this drug?

- Is there a generic version available?

DO TELL

- The names of all the drugs you are taking

- The names of all the herbs, supplements and vitamins you are taking

- If you are pregnant, trying to become pregnant or breastfeeding

- If you drink alcohol

- Any medication problems you have in addition to the ones you're being treated for

- If you experience an adverse reaction to a drug

It is important to follow your doctor's instructions for taking your medications. The chart on the following pages can help you keep track of the medications you take and when you take them. See the example below.

Drug-Usage Chart Sample

Make photocopies of this chart and use it to keep track of your medicines. Fill in the information about each drug you are taking, including those you bought over the counter. Every time you take your medicine, record it on the chart.

	MON	TUES	WED	THUR	FRI	SAT	SUN
Drug: _Paxil_ Amount in each tablet or capsule: _20 mg_ # of tablets or capsules & when to take them: _1_	8:30 a.m.	8:20 a.m.	8:30 a.m.	8:15 a.m.	8:15 a.m.	9 a.m.	9:30 a.m.

Drug-Usage Chart

Make photocopies of this chart and use it to keep track of your medicines. Fill in the information about each drug you are taking, including those you bought over the counter. Every time you take your medicine, record it on the chart.

	MON	TUES	WED	THUR	FRI	SAT	SUN
Drug: _____ Amount in each tablet or capsule: _____ # of tablets or capsules & when to take them: _____ Instructions: _____							
Drug: _____ Amount in each tablet or capsule: _____ # of tablets or capsules & when to take them: _____ Instructions: _____							
Drug: _____ Amount in each tablet or capsule: _____ # of tablets or capsules & when to take them: _____ Instructions: _____							
Drug: _____ Amount in each tablet or capsule: _____ # of tablets or capsules & when to take them: _____ Instructions: _____							

ACTIVITY

	MON	TUES	WED	THUR	FRI	SAT	SUN
Drug: _____ Amount in each tablet or capsule: _____ # of tablets or capsules & when to take them: _____ _____ Instructions: _____ _____							
Drug: _____ Amount in each tablet or capsule: _____ # of tablets or capsules & when to take them: _____ _____ Instructions: _____ _____							
Drug: _____ Amount in each tablet or capsule: _____ # of tablets or capsules & when to take them: _____ _____ Instructions: _____ _____							
Drug: _____ Amount in each tablet or capsule: _____ # of tablets or capsules & when to take them: _____ _____ Instructions: _____ _____							
Drug: _____ Amount in each tablet or capsule: _____ # of tablets or capsules & when to take them: _____ _____ Instructions: _____ _____							

Put Your Fibromyalgia on Trial

If you're frustrated with the relatively few treatment options available to people with fibromyalgia, you may want to take an active role in developing new treatments.

Consider participating in a clinical trial. Clinical trials are research studies designed to test new treatments. Not only do you get to try a treatment that may help ease your fibromyalgia symptoms, you get to try the treatment for free and may even be compensated for your participation.

Locating a study that works for you can take some legwork. The following suggestions may help you find a clinical trial near you.

- Check with your local Arthritis Foundation chapter or support group.
- Search the Internet (good sites to visit: www.centerwatch.com or www.clinicaltrials.gov).
- Scan the newspaper. Researchers often recruit participants for clinical trials via the local paper.
- Call the academic research center or teaching hospital nearest you.
- Talk to your doctor or other health-care professional.

Clearing the Fog

Many people with fibromyalgia experience unclear thinking or cognitive dysfunction. They become forgetful, lose their train of thought, forget words or mix them up. This is what is popularly known as "fibro fog." There's no known cause for it, and the only treatment for it is following some basic memory and communication tips.

Below are some common-sense pointers that can help you clear the fog. Mark those that work for you.

❑ Repeat yourself. Repeat things to yourself over and over again. Repetition will keep thoughts fresh in your mind.

❑ Write it down. Whether you write in a calendar, in a notebook or on sticky notes, if you're afraid you won't remember something, putting pen to paper can help.

❑ Pick your best time. If there is something you need to do that requires concentration and memory, such as balancing your checkbook or following a recipe, pick your best time to do it. Many people with fibromyalgia say they perform best early in the day.

❑ Get treated. Depression, pain and sleep deprivation can influence your ability to concentrate and remember. Getting your medical problems treated may indirectly help your memory.

❏ **Engage yourself.** Reading a book, seeing a play, or working a complex crossword or jigsaw puzzle can stimulate your brain and your memory.

❏ **Stay active.** Physical activity, in moderation, can increase your energy and help lift your fibro fog. Speak to your doctor or physical therapist about an exercise program that's right for you.

❏ **Explain yourself.** Explain your memory difficulties to family members and close friends. Memory problems often result from stress. Getting a little understanding from the ones you love may help.

❏ **Keep it quiet.** A radio blasting from the next room, a TV competing for your attention, or background conversation can distract your attention from the task at hand. If possible, move to a quiet place and minimize distractions when you are trying to remember.

❏ **Go slowly.** Sometimes memory problems can result from trying to do too much in too short a period of time. Break up tasks, and don't take on more than you can handle at once. Stress and fatigue will only make the situation worse.

Help for Headaches

Headaches are commonplace for nearly half of people with fibromyalgia. They can vary from mild to severe, from tension headaches to migraines. Depending on the type of headaches you get and the severity of them, your doctor can prescribe medications to help relieve the pain. There also are some nondrug strategies you can follow to prevent headaches. Here are a few:

• Keep a daily record of activities, diet, medications, sleep times and headache symptoms to target and eliminate causes of headaches. (See "Common Headache Triggers," next page.)

• Treat stress with a heating pad or ice pack before a headache begins.
• Avoid sitting or standing in one position for prolonged periods. Take frequent breaks from computer work.
• Incorporate moderate exercise into your daily routine. Gentle stretching exercises, physical therapy, massage and yoga may help.
• Consider alternative therapies, such as acupuncture, biofeedback, relaxation techniques and stress management training. (See Chapter 13 for suggested stress-management activities.)

Common Headache Triggers

The following checklist includes some possible headache triggers. Check the boxes next to the triggers that apply to you. Then go over the triggers with your doctor or other health professional so you can figure out if they are related to your headaches and you can develop a plan to control and prevent headaches.

PHYSIOLOGICAL
❏ Dieting/fasting

❏ Fatigue

❏ Hereditary predisposition

❏ Hormonal changes

❏ Irregular sleep habits

❏ Medications

❏ Menstruation

❏ Stress

ENVIRONMENTAL
❏ Altitude

❏ Cleaning compounds

❏ Lighting

❏ Noise

❏ Odors

❏ Perfume

❏ Pollution

❏ Weather changes

DIETARY
❏ Food additives (aspartame, nitrates/nitrites, yellow food coloring, MSG, tyramine)

❏ Alcohol (red wine, champagne)

❏ Caffeine (coffee, tea, cola)

❏ Cheeses

❏ Chocolate

❏ Fruits (Avocados, bananas, citrus, figs, raisins, red plums, raspberries)

❏ Pickled foods

❏ Processed or smoked meats, liver

❏ Vegetables (broad, fava and Italian green beans; snow peas; sauerkraut)

❏ Foods containing brewer's yeast, yeast extract, hydrolyzed protein extract

IBS Control

Irritable bowel syndrome (IBS) affects as many as five out of 10 people with fibromyalgia. Although IBS doesn't cause permanent harm to your intestines, the symptoms of diarrhea, constipation, abdominal cramping and bloating certainly can ruin your day.

Common triggers for IBS include poor nutrition, food and medicine sensitivity, hormone imbalances or stress. Controlling these triggers may be the first step to controlling your IBS. In addition, your doctor may prescribe medications to relieve specific symptoms. The following tips may help you control the common triggers of IBS:

- Drink plenty of water to aid digestion and avoid dehydration.

- Exercise regularly, as approved by your doctor (for example, walking). (See Chapter 6 for exercise suggestions.)

- Practice stress-reduction techniques, such as guided imagery or meditation. (See Chapter 13 for more stress-reduction exercises.)

- Eat multiple small meals rather than three large meals daily. Large meals can cause cramping and diarrhea in people with IBS.

- Use appropriate medication to control symptoms; avoid dependency on over-the-counter laxatives.

GOOD LIVING
GOOD LIVING
GOOD LIVING
GOOD LIVING
GOOD LIVING
GOOD LIVING
GOOD LIVING
GOOD LIVING
GOOD LIVING
GOOD LIVING

CHAPTER 3:

Alternative Therapies

By literal definition, one assumes *alternative therapy* means a sub-stitute therapy in place of a more traditional or mainstream Western medical therapy. However, more often today, alternative therapies are really *complementary therapies,* or unconventional ther-apies used in conjunction with more traditional treatments.

Many people with fibromyalgia rely on the added therapeutic ben-efits of alternative therapies to aid their medical treatments in easing symptoms, such as pain, fatigue and stress, and improve their overall outlook and well-being.

Which Alternative Therapies Have You Tried?

Have you tried any of the following alternative therapies to help ease the pain and other symptoms of fibromyalgia? Check the boxes of those you've tried.

To learn more about these and other alternative therapies for people with fibromyalgia, arthritis and related conditions, read *The Arthritis Foundation's Guide to Alternative Therapies* (see box, page 25).

❏ **Acupressure** The application of pressure on specific muscle sites to relieve pain and muscle spasm.

❏ **Acupuncture** Centuries-old method of pain relief used in China and introduced into Western culture in recent years that uses needles to puncture the body at sites associated with pain blockage.

❏ **Bee venom** A therapy widely used in Asia and Eastern Europe that involves the injection of bee venom into painful areas or trigger points on the body to help relieve pain.

❏ **Biofeedback** A procedure that uses electrical stimuli to increase your awareness of your body's reaction to stress and pain and to help you learn how to control your body's physical reaction.

❏ **Diet** The elimination or inclusion of certain foods into one's daily diet to relieve the symptoms of fibromyalgia.

❏ **Guided imagery** A method of managing pain and stress. Following the voice of a "guide," an audiotape or videotape, or one's own internal voice, attention is focused on a series of images that lead one's mind away from the stressor or pain.

❏ **Herbs and supplements** A common therapy for people with fibromyalgia who rely on the healing effects of natural ingredients found in herbs, minerals, enzymes and oils to ease pain, fatigue, sleeplessness, fibro fog and other symptoms.

❏ **Hypnosis** An induced sleeplike state in which you readily accept the hypnotist's suggestions.

❏ **Magnet therapy** A therapy that dates back centuries, magnets are believed to help relieve pain when worn or placed close to the body.

❏ **Massage** A technique of applying pressure, friction or vibration to the muscles by hand or using a massage appliance to stimulate circulation and produce relaxation and pain relief.

❏ **Meditation** A sustained period of deep inward thought, reflection and openness to inspiration.

❏ **Prayer** Faith in God or a higher power is not only used to comfort you and help you learn to cope with fibromyalgia, it is also believed by some to ease pain and improve health.

❏ **Relaxation** A state of release from mental or physical stress or tension.

❏ **Yoga** A system of exercises that promote control of the body and the mind.

Know Your Supplements

Herbal remedies are becoming increasingly popular with people with fibromyalgia. There are supplements available for everything from easing pain and depression to helping you lose weight and increase your energy. But with so little information available about supplements, how do you choose the right ones? Use this checklist to help you choose your supplements wisely:

❑ Have you read the label carefully? Choose products sold by large, well-known manufacturers that can be held accountable for their products. Make sure you understand the ingredient list, and if you do not, ask your pharmacist.

❑ Has the product been clinically tested? Unfortunately, not many supplements have been tested, but researchers are investigating the effects of supplements every day. Stay informed and read up on them.

❑ Is the product "standardized"? Look for "USP" on the label. This means the manufacturer followed the U.S. Pharmacopeia's standards.

❑ Have you discussed the product with your doctor and pharmacist? You should consult your doctor before trying any herbal remedy. It may counteract your prescribed treatment.

Don't Believe the Hype

Can your supplement deliver what it promises? Many supplement manufacturers make impossible claims on their labels and in their advertisements. Suspect a supplement if it:

* Comes without any directions for proper use
* Does not list contents
* Provides no information or warnings about side effects
* Claims to be based on a secret formula
* Says it cures fibromyalgia
* Cites 100-percent success

Learn More About Alternative Therapies

The Arthritis Foundation's Guide to Alternative Therapies ($24.95) offers reliable answers to your questions about nearly 90 different forms of alternative treatments, including supplements, acupuncture, tai chi, yoga, chiropractic, meditation, magnet therapy and more. To order the book, call 800/207-8633 or visit the Arthritis Foundation's online arthritis store at www.arthritis.org.

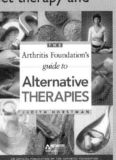

Fibromyalgia Supplement Guide

CMO

Cetyl myristoleate or cerasomal-cis-9-cetylmyristoleate

Source: A waxy substance that comes from beef tallow

Claims: Eases symptoms of RA, OA, fibromyalgia, Sjögren's syndrome and ankylosing spondylitis

How It's Used: Comes in capsules. No typical dosage. Also available in creams.

Safety/Effectiveness: Unknown. No human studies. One promising animal study for RA, but no scientific evidence so far that CMO helps with arthritis symptoms of any type.

Cautions/Side Effects/Interactions: Some instructions for taking CMO advise stopping other medications. To avoid irreversible joint damage, do not stop taking any prescription medication without talking to your doctor first. Possibility of contamination.

DHEA

Dehydroepiandrosterone

Source: A mild hormone compound produced naturally in the body to make other hormones; as a supplement, derived from chemically-treated wild yam

Claims: Relieves pain, inflammation and fatigue; used for lupus

How It's Used: Internally, in pill form.

Safety/Effectiveness: Commercial products poten-

tially unsafe, effectiveness not known. Prescription-quality DHEA may be effective as a treatment for lupus, and is under FDA review for approval as a prescription drug. In studies, a prescription grade of DHEA has allowed women to lower glucocorticoid doses. Also appeared to increase bone density.

Cautions/Side Effects/Interactions: Do not use without a prescription or a doctor's supervision. Like all hormones, DHEA can be dangerous: Possible side effects include acne, hair growth, changes in menstrual pattern, abdominal pain and hypertension. Soy might decrease its effects. If you have diabetes, DHEA can increase insulin resistance or sensitivity, so monitor blood glucose level closely. Possibility of liver damage, if you're talking azathioprine (*Imuran*) or methotrexate.

Comments: Wild yam products that claim to have "natural" DHEA don't contain any usable hormone: The pre-hormone ingredients in yam must be chemically processed before your body can use them. Do not buy DHEA off the shelf; see your doctor if you are interested in trying it.

FISH OIL

Source: Oils from cold-water fish, such as salmon, mackerel

Claims: Treats pain, stiffness,

inflammation, fatigue and depression; eases symptoms of RA, Raynaud's phenomenon, systemic lupus

How It's Used: Internally, in capsules; usual dose is about 3 grams of the active ingredients EPA and DHA. Side effects can be minimized by taking the supplements with meals and starting with low doses, increasing gradually.

Safety/Effectiveness: Several human studies show that the Omega-3 fatty acids EPA and DHA in fish oil reduce inflammation and pain of RA; also may ease symptoms of Raynaud's and may relieve depression. Likely safe and effective for RA.

Cautions/Side Effects/Interactions: Can multiply the effects of other blood thinners (such as NSAIDs and some herbs and vitamins); may also cause belching, bad breath, heartburn and nosebleeds. High doses can cause nausea and diarrhea.

Comments: Although fish oil has benefits, it takes a lot of pills to get the effects. Cold-water fish such as salmon, mackerel, tuna and halibut contain EPA and DHA, and can be beneficial if eaten two to three times a week.

GINSENG

American ginseng: Panax quinquefolius

Asian ginseng: Panax ginseng

Siberian ginseng:
Eleutherococcus senticosus

Source: The roots of two different but related plant types

Claims: Reduces fatigue; eases fibromyalgia symptoms

How It's Used: Usually taken in capsules or tablets, also available as a tea; dosage varies, but usually about 100 mg standardized extract twice a day; powdered root dosage is usually 500 mg to 1,000 mg daily.

Safety/Effectiveness: No evidence it helps for any kind of arthritis, including fibromyalgia. Animal and test tube studies suggest ginseng may benefit the immune system. But human studies are mixed, and there are none to support most claims. Generally safe when used for three months or less.

Cautions/Side Effects/Interactions: Rarely causes side effects, but can act as a mild stimulant. Women with hormone-sensitive conditions and people with hypertension should avoid ginseng. Panax ginsengs may amplify effects of glucocorticoids such as prednisone. It can change blood glucose level, so those with diabetes should use it cautiously. May increase effects of estrogen drugs. Do not take with MAO inhibitors.

Comments: This is one of the most popular and expensive supplements, but quality can vary widely.

GREEN TEA
Camellia sinensis

Source: A tea that is steamed and dried, rather than fermented like black teas

Claims: Relieves pain and inflammation

How It's Used: As a beverage, or as an extract in capsules, tablets and tinctures. Available loose and in bags for brewing. Suggested dosage is three or four cups of tea per day or the equivalent in green tea extract. Do not exceed five cups per day. A typical cup of tea has about 200 mg of polyphenols. Do not take green tea with milk, as milk may interfere with the action of the polyphenols.

Safety/Effectiveness: No human studies or evidence that green tea is effective for RA or any other kind of arthritis. In animal studies it eased arthritis-like symptoms. Green tea contains polyphenols, antioxidant compounds believed to reduce inflammation; considered safe as a beverage taken in moderate amounts.

Cautions/Side Effects/Interactions: Green tea may cause an allergic reaction. Contains caffeine; can cause stomach upset and constipation; can amplify the effects of drugs such as aspirin and acetaminophen.

Comments: Green tea has been used medicinally and as a beverage in Asia for thousands of years, and is believed to protect against cancer and other diseases. It's a healthy alternative to coffee.

KAVA KAVA
Piper methysticum

Source: The root of the kava plant

Claims: Eases pain; treats depression and anxiety

How It's Used: Usual daily dosage 140 mg to 210 mg of an ingredient called kava lactones in capsules; as drink, 1 ml to 3 ml of fresh kava.

Safety/Effectiveness: No evidence it helps with arthritis. Likely safe for short-term use; possibly unsafe in high doses or long term.

Cautions/Side Effects/Interactions: Can cause upset stomach, headache and dizziness. Heavy use of kava may impair thinking and activities that require concentration, such as driving; do not mix with tranquilizers or drugs, such as sleeping medications or alcohol.

MAGNESIUM

Use: To relieve pain and inflammation; to ease fibromyalgia and chronic fatigue symptoms

Scientific Evidence: A placebo-controlled study of a magnesium and malic acid combination product found it eased pain and boosted energy in 24 women with fibromyalgia.

Fibromyalgia Supplement Guide (continued)

Dosage: Comes in many forms, and usually is combined with malic acid for treatment of fibromyalgia. Suggested daily dose: malic acid, 1,200 mg to 2,400 mg; magnesium, 300 mg to 600 mg, divided into several doses. Magnesium RDA is 320 mg for women, 420 mg for men.

Cautions/Comments: Chronic fatigue symptoms are connected to low magnesium levels, and supplements have been shown to improve those symptoms. Can interact with blood pressure medication; may cause loose stools; do not use if you have kidney problems because it can cause kidney failure; may cause nausea, vomiting, diarrhea, stomach irritation. Food sources include nuts, grains and whole foods.

MELATONIN
N-acetyl-5-methoxytryptamine

Source: A natural hormone made in the pineal gland deep in the brain; supplements are usually synthetic (made from chemicals), but some come from animal pineal tissue

Claims: Boosts the immune system; cures sleep problems; prevents osteoporosis

How It's Used: Usual dose is 0.3 mg to 3 mg taken a few hours before bedtime.

Safety/Effectiveness: Decreased melatonin levels have been found in insomniacs and in patients with sleep disorders related to other condi-

tions, such as fibromyalgia and depression. Studies show melatonin appears to boost the immune system and help regulate sleep. Possibly safe and effective as a sleep aid for people without any medical conditions. Possibly unsafe for those with autoimmune diseases including lupus.

Cautions/Side Effects/ Interactions: Those with autoimmune diseases, including lupus, or depression should not take melatonin. Since melatonin is a hormone, it can have far-reaching and unpredictable effects.

Comments: A controlled-release product (not available in the United States) is undergoing trials as a prescription drug for use in Canada and Europe.

SAM-e
S-adenosylmethionine

Source: Naturally occurring compound produced from methionine, a sulfur-containing amino acid, and adenosine triphosphate (ATP); supplements are made from fermented yeast or synthesized

Claims: Relieves symptoms of OA and fibromyalgia; treats depression; eases pain and stiffness

How It's Used: Internally, in tablets. In OA studies, SAM-e was taken in doses of 200 mg to 400 mg three times per day. For fibromyalgia, 800 mg per day is typical, increasing

dosage gradually from 200 mg per day. For depression, 1,600 mg per day is recommended.

Safety/Effectiveness: Several human studies show SAM-e relieves OA pain and other symptoms as well as NSAIDs do, without side effects. Some studies show it relieved pain and other fibromyalgia symptoms. Other studies show it as effective as tricyclic antidepressants without the side effects. Likely safe and effective for OA pain and short-term depression.

Cautions/Side Effects/ Interactions: May cause nausea or upset stomach; side effects more common with higher doses; might interact with certain anti-depressants; do not take SAM-e if you are seriously depressed or have bipolar disorder (manic-depression): It may contribute to a manic state.

Comments: SAM-e is expensive and not very stable, so the product you buy might not have any active ingredients. Look for products that are packaged to be air- and light-proof and that are in the form of 1,4 butanedisulfonate, which is more stable. SAM-e is a prescription drug in Europe.

ST. JOHN'S WORT
Hypericum perforatum

Source: A small yellow flower that grows wild throughout Europe and the United States, primarily in northern California and Oregon

Claims: Acts as "natural *Prozac*" for depression; may also have anti-inflammatory effects

How It's Used: Internally, in pills, teas and tincture. Dose in some clinical trials is 300 mg three times daily of an extract standardized to 0.3 percent hypericin. One cup of the tea is usually taken one to three times per day. Oily topical solution used for muscle pain to relieve inflammation.

Safety/Effectiveness: St. John's wort contains hypericin and hyperforin, chemicals that raise the levels of serotonin in the brain. Serotonin levels are known to be low in people who are depressed and in those with fibromyalgia. Studies have shown St. John's wort can relieve mild depression about as well as tricyclic and SSRI antidepressants. Generally safe and effective for mild depression. Needs to be taken for several weeks to feel the effect. However, a large new study found it not effective for serious depression.

Cautions/Side Effects/Interactions: May increase sensitivity to sunlight and risk of sunburn in fair-skinned people. Can block the effects of drugs, including oral contraceptives, HIV medications, tricyclic antidepressants, cyclosporin, several heart drugs and warfarin. It can amplify the effects of many drugs, such as MAO inhibitors, SSRI antidepressants, tranquilizers, alcohol and many herbs. Do not take if you are severely depressed, or if you have bipolar disorder (manic depression). If your symptoms do not improve within two months, talk to your doctor about a stronger antidepressant. Side effects may include insomnia (which can be avoided by taking St. John's wort in the morning or decreasing the dose), restlessness, anxiety, irritability, stomach pain, fatigue, dry mouth, dizziness and headache.

Comments: Widely prescribed in Europe, St. John's wort is one of the top-selling supplements in the United States as well. Use with care because it has many drug and herb interactions.

VALERIAN

Valeriana officinalis

Source: The root of a pink flower that grows wild throughout the Americas, Europe and Asia

Claims: Treats insomnia and muscle and joint pain

How It's Used: Internally, usually taken as an herbal extract in capsules or tea about an hour before bedtime. Also comes in a tincture or in combination with other hops and herbs. The tea is prepared by steeping 2 grams to 3 grams of the root in boiling water. Typical dose is one cup of the tea taken one to several times per day; the maximum dose is 15 grams of the root per day. Externally, can be used in a bath for restlessness and sleep disorders.

Safety/Effectiveness: Several studies show it might be an effective alternative to conventional sleep drugs. No evidence it eases other arthritis-related symptoms. Probably safe when used short term, and may be effective for insomnia.

Cautions/Side Effects/Interactions: No known serious side effects. Do not drink alcohol and take valerian, or take with other sleep aids or tranquilizers, as it increases the effects. May cause morning drowsiness; after extended use, reduce dose gradually. Don't drive or perform other activities requiring alertness after taking.

Comments: Approved by German health officials as a mild sleep aid and sedative. The root has been a popular treatment of insomnia and anxiety for centuries in other countries.

Ten Supplements To Avoid

SUPPLEMENT	CLAIM	WHY YOU SHOULD AVOID IT
ARNICA *Arnica Montana*	Relieves aches; an anti-inflammatory and immune system enhancer.	Can cause miscarriages, allergic reactions, paralysis, heart palpitations, death.
ACONITE *Aconitum napellus*	Eases joint inflammation, gout, RA.	Is a fast-acting poison that affects the heart.
ADRENAL, SPLEEN, THYMUS EXTRACTS	Helps fatigue, and relieves stress and inflammation.	Derived from animal organs. FDA warns organs could possibly be contaminated.
AUTUMN CROCUS *Colchicum autumnale*	Lessens gout attacks and eases general arthritis pain.	Is a potential poison. Taken only as a prescription drug (colchicine) under a doctor's supervision.
5-HTP *5-hydroxytryptophan*	Helps fibromyalgia, sleep disorders and depression.	Associated with eosinophilia myalgia, a serious illness that causes severe rashes, acute pain and other symptoms.
GHB *Gamma-hydroxybutyrate*	Helps fibromyalgia, sleep disorders, pain and fatigue.	Known as the "date rape" drug. May cause coma or death. Should be used only with doctor's supervision.
GBL *Gamma-butyrolactone*	Helps fibromyalgia, sleep problems, depression, claims to "improve sexual and athletic performance and health."	Has been linked to deaths, coma and seizures.
L-TRYPTOPHAN	Eases sleep disorders and depression.	Is illegal in the United States. Associated with eosinophilia myalgia, a serious illness that causes severe rashes, acute pain and other symptoms.
CHAPARRAL	Reduces inflammation.	Is poisonous. May cause hepatitis, kidney and liver damage.
KOMBUCHA TEA	Helps "rheumatism" and eases pain.	Has high risk of contamination with anthrax and other bacteria.

Be Label Savvy

Since 1999, the FDA has required manufacturers to create supplement labels that are easier to read and understand.

So before you even consider buying a remedy, spend some time perusing those labels. Bring a magnifying glass if you have to, to read the "fine print." Compare the listing of ingredients to the package's claims. Check dosage, strength and price on various products with the same ingredients. Remember that supplements are not regulated like other drugs – the FDA does not test products before sale, regulate how they are manufactured or even require proof that the supplement contains or does what it says it's supposed to. The FDA does, however, state that manufacturers and marketers can't make medical claims without a disclaimer that states they do not have FDA approval.

Once you turn over that bottle, here's what you'll see on the Supplement Facts panel:

- Serving size or dose suggested by manufacturer

- Active ingredients, with amount per dose

- Percent Daily Value (DV), or the percentage each ingredient provides of the recommended daily intake (RDI). If the RDI hasn't been determined, you will see an asterisk.

- Inactive ingredients, which are substances used in manufacturing. These components help process and package the active ingredients, hold pills or ointments together, or make the product easier to swallow or apply. Although these substances have little or no effect, they still could cause an allergic reaction, so be aware of them.

- Instructions for use of the product

- Storage information. Many products lose potency when not stored properly.

- Expiration date

- Cautions, including interactions, allergic reactions and other possible problems

- The manufacturer's or distributor's name, address and zip code

- Manufacturer's batch or lot number, which allows a product to be traced. If you have any side effects, you will want to give this information to the FDA.

- Disclaimer. This is required if health claims are made.

- "USP" symbol, which indicates the product meets U.S. Pharmacopeia standards for quality, strength, purity, packaging and labeling. Although you'll want to purchase products with the USP mark, it does not mean the product has government approval for safety or effectiveness.

Supplement Diary

Photocopy this diary and use it to record any herbs, supplements, vitamins and minerals you are taking.

Treatment: _____

Used for: _____

Amount taken: _____

When taken: _____

Special instructions: _____

_____

Date started: _____ Date stopped: _____

Possible side effects/drug interactions: _____

_____

Notes: _____

Treatment: _____

Used for: _____

Amount taken: _____

When taken: _____

Special instructions: _____

_____

Date started: _____ Date stopped: _____

Possible side effects/drug interactions: _____

_____

Notes: _____

Treatment: _____

Used for: _____

Amount taken: _____

When taken: _____

Special instructions: _____

_____

Date started: _____ Date stopped: _____

Possible side effects/drug interactions: _____

_____

Notes: _____

Treatment: _____

Used for: _____

Amount taken: _____

When taken: _____

Special instructions: _____

_____

Date started: _____ Date stopped: _____

Possible side effects/drug interactions: _____

_____

Notes: _____

Treatment: _____

Used for: _____

Amount taken: _____

When taken: _____

Special instructions: _____

_____

Date started: _____ Date stopped: _____

Possible side effects/drug interactions: _____

_____

Notes: _____

Treatment: _____

Used for: _____

Amount taken: _____

When taken: _____

Special instructions: _____

_____

Date started: _____ Date stopped: _____

Possible side effects/drug interactions: _____

_____

Notes: _____

Talking to Your Doctor About Alternative Therapies

Some doctors are reticent about recommending alternative therapies to their patients with fibromyalgia for one simple reason: They often know little about alternative therapies. Doctors rely on medical literature to keep them up-to-date on the latest treatments, and, unfortunately, there are few published studies that discuss alternative therapies.

However, you and your doctor can discuss alternative therapies and share ideas and suggestions. Together, you can create a treatment plan that includes both traditional and alternative therapies.

The following tips can help you open the doors of communicating with your doctor about alternative therapies. The "Ask the Doctor" worksheet on page 37 can help you prepare for your next appointment.

• Be candid about any alternative medicines you are already taking. Your doctor can't help you or protect you if he or she doesn't know the whole story.

• Tell your doctor about any therapies you are considering, and share what you have been reading or hearing about various therapies.

• Ask your doctor what he or she knows about any therapy you are considering, especially any possible dangers, such as drug interactions with medications you are taking. Also ask your doctor to refer you to an established practitioner, or to write you a prescription for the alternative therapy. That will improve your chances for insurance coverage.

• If your doctor objects to the treatments you propose, find out why. Although doctors are increasingly open to combining traditional and complementary medicine, not all of them favor this approach.

GOOD LIVING
GOOD LIVING
GOOD LIVING
GOOD LIVING
GOOD LIVING
GOOD LIVING
GOOD LIVING
GOOD LIVING
GOOD LIVING
GOOD LIVING

CHAPTER 4:

Medical Managers

It takes the help of an understanding doctor to develop a successful treatment plan. That is why it is important not only to find the right doctor, but also to be sure you are making the most of your appointments together.

Only you know how you feel or where you hurt, so it is up to you to keep track of your pain and symptoms. The worksheets in this chapter will help you get organized.

Doctor Visit Prep

Having a condition that varies so significantly from person to person, you need to be the watchdog for your individual mix of symptoms. This is particularly important when you see the doctor.

Doctors' visits are the time for you to discuss your condition and symptoms and to go over treatments. You also may have questions and concerns that you'd like to discuss. To be sure that you get the most out of your doctor's appointment, try using the worksheets on the following pages to prepare for your next appointment.

For a who's who list of your health-care team, see Chapter 4 of *The Arthritis Foundation's Guide to Good Living With Fibromyalgia*.

Choose Your Doctor Wisely

Finding the right doctor may be one of the most important things you can do to help you learn to manage your fibromyalgia. Whether you are looking for a general practitioner or a specialist, here are several tips for choosing the best doctor for you:

ASK YOUR FRIENDS. Do you have friends with fibromyalgia who are happy with their doctors? Get a referral. You also can contact your local Arthritis Foundation chapter for a referral list (call 800/283-7800 or visit www.arthritis.org to find a chapter near you).

SHOP AROUND. Don't simply choose the first name on a list. Interview a few doctors to determine their knowledge of, interest in and attitude toward fibromyalgia.

LOOK AT THE BIG PICTURE. A doctor in a small, single practice may be nice, but one working in a university center or large medical practice has the opportunity to interact with more colleagues, residents, students and patients.

LOOK FOR A LISTENER. Find a doctor who will listen to you and allow you to participate in your treatment decisions.

ACTIVITY

"Ask the Doctor"

Photocopy these worksheets and use them as you prepare for your doctor's visits.

Complete this part before the visit:

1. What is the main reason I am going to the doctor?

2. Is there anything else that concerns me about my health or treatment (e.g., effect of fibromyalgia on work, family or mood; problems following the recommended treatment plan)?

_____ Yes _____ No

3. What do I want the doctor to do today?

4. The symptoms that bother me the most are ... (What? Where? When did they start? Do they change over time? How long do they last?). NOTE: bring copies of any completed self-monitoring forms/diaries.

5. What medications (prescriptions and over-the-counter) am I taking regularly? (List name(s) and dosage, or take the bottles to your appointment.)

6. What are my goals for treatment (what I want or expect to get out of treatment)?

7. Prepare and prioritize a list of questions to give the doctor early in the visit.

8. Do I need Medicare, Medicaid or other insurance cards/forms today?

_____ Yes _____ No

"Ask the Doctor" (continued)

Questions to ask your doctor during the visit:

1. What is happening to me? How is my fibromyalgia likely to affect me?

   _____

2. What are the results of my tests, and what do they mean? May I have a copy of the results?

   _____

3. Why do I need the lab tests or X-rays that you are recommending today?

   _____

4. Are there any risks from these tests?

   _____

5. When should I call for the results?

   _____

6. What should I do at home (diet, activity, treatment options, special instructions, medications, precautions, etc.)?

   _____

a. What are the benefits, costs and drawbacks (or risks) for each option for treatment?

   _____

b. How and how often do I take the treatment?

   _____

c. How long should I give it a try?

   _____

7. When should I call if my condition doesn't get better and the treatment does not seem to be working? What additional symptoms would warrant my calling before my next scheduled visit?

   _____

8. When should I return for another visit?

   _____

ACTIVITY

Medication questions:

1. What is the name of the drug? _____

2. What are the purpose and benefits of this drug?

   _____

3. How quickly does it work? How long should I take this drug?

   _____

4. What are the possible side effects or drawbacks to the drug?

   _____

   a. When should I contact you about side effects?

   _____

   b. What can I do to prevent or deal with the side effects or drawbacks?

   _____

5. Is it all right to take the drug with other drugs (such as cold, sinus, allergy, pain medicines) I am taking? _____ Yes _____ No
   If not, what drugs should I avoid?

6. When is the best time to take the drug? Before, with or after meals?

7. What should I do if I forget to take my medicine?

   _____

8. Are there any changes I should make in my diet? _____ Yes _____ No
   If so, what? _____

   a. Can I drink alcohol while taking this drug? _____ Yes _____ No

   b. Are there any other restrictions? _____ Yes _____ No
   If so, what? _____

9. Should I avoid driving while taking this drug? _____ Yes _____ No

10. Is a generic drug available? _____ Yes _____ No

ACTIVITY

Get Organized

Fibro fog or not, keeping track of all of your medications, health-care providers, medical history and health insurance information can be daunting. Use the following pages to keep track of your personal health-care record.

HEALTH-CARE TEAM INFORMATION

Record the names and contact information for your health-care team, including physicians, physical therapists, counselors and any other specialists you visit.

Name

Specialty

Practice

Address

City	State	Zip

Phone	After hours

Fax

Office hours

Nurse/Office manager

Accepts my insurance plan?

Name

Specialty

Practice

Address

City	State	Zip

Phone	After hours

Fax

Office hours

Nurse/Office manager

Accepts my insurance plan?

Name

Specialty

Practice

Address

City   State   Zip

Phone   After hours

Fax

Office hours

Nurse/Office manager

Accepts my insurance plan?

Name

Specialty

Practice

Address

City   State   Zip

Phone   After hours

Fax

Office hours

Nurse/Office manager

Accepts my insurance plan?

Name

Specialty

Practice

Address

City   State   Zip

Phone   After hours

Fax

Office hours

Nurse/Office manager

Accepts my insurance plan?

INSURANCE PROVIDER INFORMATION

List information about your health insurance policies.

Company

Policy holder

Policy number

Address

City	State	Zip

Phone

Fax

Contact

Payment Information

Company

Policy holder

Policy number

Address

City	State	Zip

Phone

Fax

Contact

Payment Information

Company

Policy holder

Policy number

Address

City	State	Zip

Phone

Fax

Contact

Payment Information

Company

Policy holder

Policy number

Address

City   State   Zip

Phone

Fax

Contact

Payment Information

Company

Policy holder

Policy number

Address

City   State   Zip

Phone

Fax

Contact

Payment Information

Company

Policy holder

Policy number

Address

City   State   Zip

Phone

Fax

Contact

Payment Information

HOSPITALS AND HEALTH-CARE FACILITIES

Record contact information for hospitals, clinics, rehab centers and other facilities you use.

Name

Address

City   State   Zip

Phone

Emergency number

Fax

Name

Address

City   State   Zip

Phone

Emergency number

Fax

Name

Address

City   State   Zip

Phone

Emergency number

Fax

Name

Address

City   State   Zip

Phone

Emergency number

Fax

Name

Address

City   State   Zip

Phone

Emergency number

Fax

Name

Address

City   State   Zip

Phone

Emergency number

Fax

Name

Address

City   State   Zip

Phone

Emergency number

Fax

Name

Address

City   State   Zip

Phone

Emergency number

Fax

PHARMACY INFORMATION

List information about the pharmacies you use.

Name   Hours of operation

Pharmacist

Address

City   State   Zip

Phone

Fax

Accepts my insurance plan?

Name   Hours of operation

Pharmacist

Address

City   State   Zip

Phone

Fax

Accepts my insurance plan?

Name   Hours of operation

Pharmacist

Address

City   State   Zip

Phone

Fax

Accepts my insurance plan?

Name   Hours of operation

Pharmacist

Address

City   State   Zip

Phone

Fax

Accepts my insurance plan?

PERSONAL MEDICAL HISTORY

Record information about your personal medical history.

Blood Type: ❑ A ❑ B ❑ AB ❑ O ❑ Positive ❑ Negative

Notes:

Allergies (foods, animal hair, medications, insect bites, etc.)

Vaccinations

TYPE	DATE

CHILDHOOD ILLNESSES AND DISEASES

Include major illnesses you had as a child, such as measles, chickenpox, juvenile arthritis, etc.

ILLNESS	DATE

Notes:

ADULT ILLNESSES AND DISEASES

Here, list other major illnesses you've had as an adult, such as rheumatoid arthritis, Lyme disease or heart disease.

ILLNESS	DATE

Notes:

OTHER MEDICAL CONDITIONS

List other conditions you have, such as high blood pressure or chronic back pain.

CONDITION	DATE

Notes:

FAMILY HISTORY OF ILLNESSES AND DISEASES

Use this section to record information about illnesses of close family members, such as parents or siblings.

ILLNESS	DATE

Notes:

SURGERIES

Use this space to record information about your surgical history.	
TYPE	DATE

LABORATORY TESTS

(Including X-rays, bone scans, blood work)
Note: If you have lab tests frequently to monitor a medication you're taking, you may not need to record each test. Instead, you may want to record them periodically to show changes or trends.

TEST	DATE	RESULT

LABORATORY TESTS (CONTINUED)

(Including X-rays, bone scans, blood work)
Note: If you have lab tests frequently to monitor a medication you're taking, you may not need to record each test. Instead, you may want to record them periodically to show changes or trends.

TEST	DATE	RESULT

Notes:

MEDICATIONS – PRESCRIPTIONS

List all prescription drugs you take.

Medication

Dosage

Prescribed by

When taken

Precautions

Date started

Date stopped

Possible side effects/drug interactions

Medication

Dosage

Prescribed by

When taken

Precautions

Date started

Date stopped

Possible side effects/drug interactions

Medication

Dosage

Prescribed by

When taken

Precautions

Date started

Date stopped

Possible side effects/drug interactions

MEDICATIONS – PRESCRIPTIONS (CONTINUED)

List all prescription drugs you take.

Medication

Dosage

Prescribed by

When taken

Precautions

Date started

Date stopped

Possible side effects/drug interactions

Medication

Dosage

Prescribed by

When taken

Precautions

Date started

Date stopped

Possible side effects/drug interactions

Medication

Dosage

Prescribed by

When taken

Precautions

Date started

Date stopped

Possible side effects/drug interactions

Medication

Dosage

Prescribed by

When taken

Precautions

Date started

Date stopped

Possible side effects/drug interactions

Medication

Dosage

Prescribed by

When taken

Precautions

Date started

Date stopped

Possible side effects/drug interactions

Medication

Dosage

Prescribed by

When taken

Precautions

Date started

Date stopped

Possible side effects/drug interactions

MEDICATIONS – OVER-THE-COUNTER

List over-the-counter drugs you take, such as pain relievers or antacids.

Medication

Used for

Amount taken

How often

Precautions

Possible side effects/drug interactions

Medication

Used for

Amount taken

How often

Precautions

Possible side effects/drug interactions

Medication

Used for

Amount taken

How often

Precautions

Possible side effects/drug interactions

Medication

Used for

Amount taken

How often

Precautions

Possible side effects/drug interactions

Medication

Used for

Amount taken

How often

Precautions

Possible side effects/drug interactions

Medication

Used for

Amount taken

How often

Precautions

Possible side effects/drug interactions

Medication

Used for

Amount taken

How often

Precautions

Possible side effects/drug interactions

Medication

Used for

Amount taken

How often

Precautions

Possible side effects/drug interactions

OTHER THERAPIES

List other therapies you use, such as physical therapy, acupuncture or massage.

Therapy

Use

Amount

How Often

Other Instructions

Precautions

Therapy

Use

Amount

How Often

Other Instructions

Precautions

Therapy

Use

Amount

How Often

Other Instructions

Precautions

Therapy

Use

Amount

How Often

Other Instructions

Precautions

Therapy

Use

Amount

How Often

Other Instructions

Precautions

Therapy

Use

Amount

How Often

Other Instructions

Precautions

Therapy

Use

Amount

How Often

Other Instructions

Precautions

Therapy

Use

Amount

How Often

Other Instructions

Precautions

OTHER THERAPIES (CONTINUED)

List other therapies you use, such as physical therapy, acupuncture or massage.

Therapy

Use

Amount

How Often

Other Instructions

Precautions

Therapy

Use

Amount

How Often

Other Instructions

Precautions

Therapy

Use

Amount

How Often

Other Instructions

Precautions

Record Your Health

The Arthritis Foundation's *Health Organizer* ($14.95) is a spiral-bound, tabbed journal that helps you track your disease activity and keep track of all of your important health documents. You can share information from your *Health Organizer* with your doctor to make sure you are getting the best treatment possible.

To order your copy, call 800/207-8633 or visit www.arthritis.org.

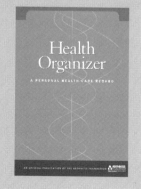

GOOD LIVING
GOOD LIVING
GOOD LIVING
GOOD LIVING
GOOD LIVING
GOOD LIVING
GOOD LIVING
GOOD LIVING
GOOD LIVING

GOOD LIVING
GOOD LIVING
GOOD LIVING
GOOD LIVING
GOOD LIVING
GOOD LIVING
GOOD LIVING
GOOD LIVING

CHAPTER 5:

Managing Your Life

You can't change the fact that you have fibromyalgia or that there will be good days and bad days. But you can change how you let fibromyalgia affect your life. Don't let your condition rule your daily activities. Taking charge of your health and finding balance between the things you love to do and the rest you need will help you achieve good living with fibromyalgia.

Do You Have the Keys To Good Living?

Maintaining a satisfying and healthy life with fibromyalgia can be trying and usually requires you to put mind over matter. Having the keys to good living can help. Place a check beside the techniques you are using to achieve good living.

❑ Optimism. Is the glass half-full or half-empty? Do you have a positive outlook? Do you believe in positive thinking?

❑ Humor. Is laughter the best medicine for you? Do you smile often?

❑ Sense of Purpose. Do you believe in yourself and that you have worth?

❑ Sense of Control. Do you feel that you are in control of your life choices, or do you feel helpless from your fibromyalgia and other life challenges?

❑ Social Support. Do you have the support and understanding of your family and friends? Do you have a support network you can turn to during trying times?

❑ Positive Self-Image. Do you like yourself?

Read more about the keys to good living in *The Arthritis Foundation's Guide to Good Living With Fibromyalgia*, Chapter 5.

Balancing Act

Another way to achieve good living is to ensure that you are balancing all the important things in your life, such as your personal relationships, work, hobbies and health.

Use the activity on the opposite page to determine how balanced your life is and which areas of your life need to be addressed. Then complete the worksheets that follow to help you learn to balance your activities and achieve "good living."

ACTIVITY

Targeting Your Time

Instructions: Read the names of each of the 12 activities listed in the wedges of the circle below. Think about how satisfied you are with the time you now spend on each activity. Color in the part of the wedge for each activity that best describes how that activity fits into your life. For example, if you are satisfied with time spent on an activity, color the center part of the wedge, in the "OK" section. Otherwise, indicate by coloring whether you "need less" or "need more" of the activity, or if the activity is "not important" in your life.

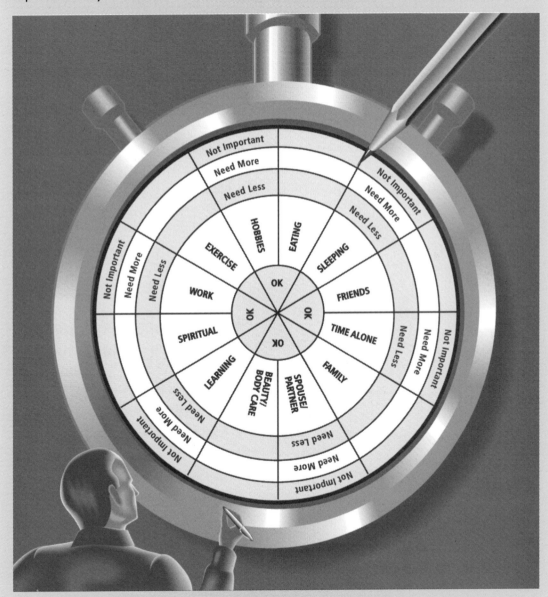

Things You Love To Do

Photocopy this worksheet and write down as many activities as possible that bring you enjoyment and happiness. In the "Rank Top Five" column, indicate by number those five activities that you enjoy the most. In the "Last Time" column, indicate how long it has been since you engaged in each of your top five activities. If you haven't done any of these activities in a long time, consider ways you can incorporate those activities more frequently into your busy life.

		Rank Top Five	Last Time
1			
2			
3			
4			
5			
6			
7			
8			
9			
10			
11			
12			
13			
14			

The Best of Me

Photocopy this worksheet and list at least 10 qualities or aspects that make you unique, that you like or admire about yourself and/or that make you attractive (include at least one or two physical attributes). Complete your list with the "Things You Like to Do." Are you doing all the activities that can make you feel best?

1

2

3

4

5

6

7

8

9

10

Tips for Good Living Every Day With Fibromyalgia

Even though you may have achieved "good living" with fibromyalgia, there may still be some everyday chores you have difficulty performing. The following tips offer you some useful help for tackling everyday tasks.

AT HOME

- Sit while you wash dishes. Place a high chair or stool near the sink so you won't have to stoop.
- Consider your time and energy when you shop or run errands. Is driving an extra 15 minutes to a discount store really worth saving 50 cents on light bulbs? Your time and energy are at least as valuable as gasoline. Keep shopping short and simple.
- Learn to make "one-pot" meals to save the time and effort of cleaning a number of dishes. Stews, pasta dishes or chicken cooked with vegetables in a foil, disposable pan or oven-baking bag can make easy meals with limited cleanup.
- Pack children's lunches the evening before, or pack several days' worth at once. Store these meals in paper sacks in the refrigerator if the items are perishable. Advance preparation cuts down on morning rush.
- Store, reheat and serve leftovers in the same microwave-safe dish so you don't have to transfer food from one dish to another, and so you don't have to wash several dishes. A dinner bowl covered with plastic wrap takes up as much space in your refrigerator as a rubber-topped storage container, and it keeps food fresh.

AT WORK

- Use coffee breaks for short walks around the office. It's important to stretch your legs and joints when your job requires hours of sitting.
- Discuss with your supervisor the possibility of adjusting your work schedule. You may be able to come to work later and leave later, allowing you extra time in the morning to take a warm bath or to practice stretching exercises.
- Alternate light and heavy tasks, doing the toughest jobs when you're feeling best.
- When using a computer, make sure you have a comfortable chair with good low-back support and arm rests. Position your wrists so that they are in line with your forearms. Lean forward at your hips instead of bending at the waist or neck.

AT PLAY

- Make time for exercise, even when you're on vacation. You will have more energy for sightseeing, and you'll keep your muscles and joints from getting stiff while sitting on tour buses or visiting museums.
- People with fibromyalgia may have problems with sling-style baby carriers, particularly if they have tender-point pain in

their shoulder. A hand-held model or folding stroller may be preferable.

- Your joints may become stiff during a long movie. Get to the theater early so you can choose an aisle seat or a handicapped-accessible seat that allows you to stretch your legs periodically.

- When traveling, use a small compartmented pill container to organize your daily medications. Keep the container in your purse, carry-on bag or suit pocket where you won't lose it and can access it easily during your trip.

- Hiking can be an enjoyable and leisurely form of exercise. Investigate any hiking trails before you embark on your hike. Avoid trails with any uneven, slippery footing, steep inclines or any trails that require you to climb using your hands. Pick an easy beginner's trail that is well-marked. Hike with friends – never alone – and bring a cellular phone and identification card with you.

AT REST

- A warm bath can be a great place to relax. Make time for your daily soak, whether in the morning to loosen stiff joints before your day, or in the evening to relax you before you sleep or have sex.

- Establish a regular sleeping schedule. Your body will be more rested and function better if you are not sleeping late one day and forcing yourself to get up very early the next morning. It's important to stick to a regular bedtime and waking time, even on weekends.

- Wear comfortable clothing when you relax. When you come home from work, remove your work clothes or any clothing that is constraining or tight. Warm-up suits, sweatshirts, sweaters and elastic-waist pants are good clothes for relaxation time.

- Your bedroom should be a place for rest and relaxation. Don't sit on the bed to do your paperwork, writing or household chores. Save the bedroom for sleeping, sex and resting. Beds should not be used as desks, as they don't provide proper back support or an appropriately positioned writing surface.

- While you're watching TV, get off the couch and walk around about once every 30 minutes – perhaps in between your favorite shows or during commercial breaks – to keep joints from stiffening. Don't just walk to the refrigerator and back.

Want More Tips?

Pick up a copy of *The Arthritis Foundation's Tips for Good Living with Arthritis* ($9.95), which includes more than 700 suggestions for daily living with arthritis and related conditions. Read hundreds of practical, tried-and-true strategies for simplifying your life at home, at work and at play.

To order, call 800/207-8633 or visit www.arthritis.org.

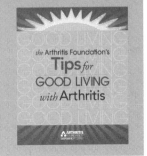

GOOD LIVING
GOOD LIVING
GOOD LIVING
GOOD LIVING
GOOD LIVING
GOOD LIVING
GOOD LIVING
GOOD LIVING
GOOD LIVING

CHAPTER 6:

Get Moving

Exercise may seem like the last thing your aching, tired muscles need, but it is, in fact, one of the best things you can do for your fibromyalgia. Exercise not only will help strengthen your muscles, give you more flexibility and improve your cardiovascular health, it may decrease your fatigue, help you sleep at night and relieve stress.

If you are worried about where to begin, the activities and exercises in this chapter will help you get started on an exercise program.

Why Exercise?

Study after study has shown that exercise can decrease pain and improve symptoms of fibromyalgia. Endorphins – your body's natural pain relievers – aren't the only benefit. Exercise can empower you to take charge of your health and control how you feel.

Why do you want to exercise? Place a check next to the benefit(s) of exercise that you hope to achieve. Exercise can:

❑ Keep my body from becoming too stiff

❑ Keep my muscles strong

❑ Keep my bone and cartilage tissue strong and healthy

❑ Improve my ability to do daily activities

❑ Give me more energy

❑ Help me sleep better

❑ Control my weight

❑ Improve my cardiovascular health

❑ Provide an outlet for stress and tension

❑ Decrease depression and anxiety

❑ Release endorphins

❑ Improve my self-esteem

❑ Provide a sense of well-being

Get Started

Range-of-motion and strengthening exercises should be an essential part of your exercise regimen. They reduce stiffness and increase joint flexibility and muscle strength. Try to work the following exercises into your warm-up or cool-down routine. Choose the exercises that are best for you, avoiding those that strain already painful areas.

These exercises have been excerpted from the Arthritis Foundation's PACE (People with Arthritis Can Exercise) program. There are PACE exercise videos for any level of fitness. To purchase copies of the PACE videos, call 800/207-8633 or shop online at www.arthritis.org.

NECK EXERCISES

Purpose: Increase neck range of motion; relax neck and shoulder muscles; improve posture.

Precautions: Do these exercises slowly and smoothly. If you feel dizzy, stop the exercise. If you have had neck problems, check with your doctor before doing these exercises.

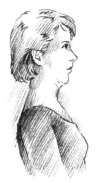
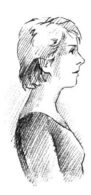
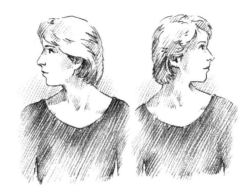

CHIN TUCKS

Pull your chin back as if to make a double chin. Keep your head straight – don't look down. Hold three seconds. Then raise your neck straight up as if someone was pulling straight up on your hair.

HEAD TURNS (ROTATION)

Turn your head to look over your shoulder. Hold three seconds. Return to the center and then turn to look over your other shoulder. Hold three seconds. Repeat.

SHOULDER EXERCISES

Purpose: Increase mobility of the shoulder girdle (the bony structure that supports your upper limbs); strengthen muscles that raise shoulders; relax neck and shoulder muscles.

Precautions: If the exercise increases pain, stop and consult with your physician.

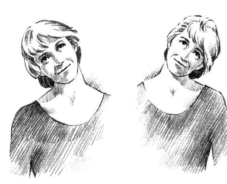
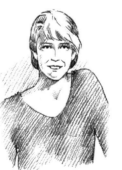
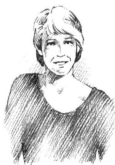

HEAD TILTS

Focus on an object in front of you. Tilt your head sideways toward your right shoulder. Hold three seconds. Return to the center, and tilt toward your left shoulder. Hold three seconds. Do not twist head but continue to look forward. Do not raise your shoulder toward your ear.

SHOULDER SHRUGS (ELEVATION)

(A) Raise one shoulder, lower it. Then raise the other shoulder; be sure the first shoulder is completely relaxed and lowered before raising the other.

(B) Raise both shoulders up toward the ears. Hold three seconds. Relax. Concentrate on completely relaxing shoulders as they come down. Do not tilt the head or body in either direction. Do not hunch your shoulders forward or pinch shoulder blades together.

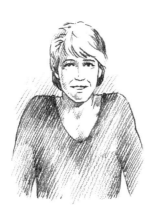 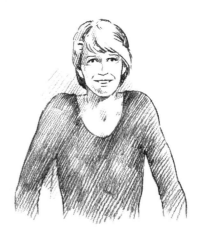

SHOULDER CIRCLES

Lift both shoulders up; move them forward, then down and back in a circling motion. Then lift both shoulders up; move them backward, then down and forward in a circling motion.

ARM EXERCISES (SHOULDERS AND ELBOWS)

Purpose: Increase shoulder and/or elbow motion; strengthen shoulder and/or elbow muscles; relax neck and shoulder muscles; improve posture.

Precautions: If you have had shoulder or elbow surgery, check with your surgeon before doing these exercises. These exercises are not advised for people with significant shoulder joint damage, such as unstable joints or total cuff tears.

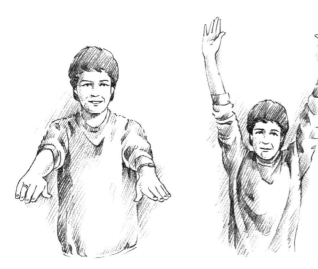

FORWARD ARM REACH

Raise one or both arms forward and upward as high as possible. Return to your starting position.

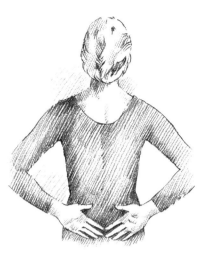 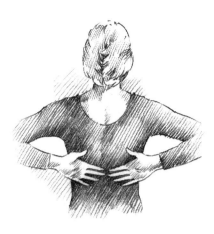

SELF BACK RUB (INTERNAL ROTATION)

While seated, slide a few inches forward from the back of your chair. Sit up as straight as possible; do not round your shoulders. Place the back of your hands on your lower back. Slowly move them upward until you feel a stretch in your shoulders. Hold three seconds, then slide your hands back down. You can use one hand to help the other. Move within the limits of your pain. Do not force.

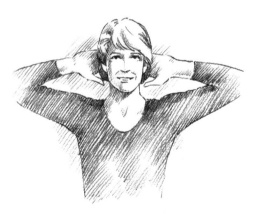 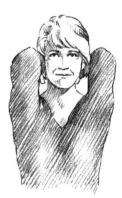

SHOULDER ROTATOR

Sit or stand as straight as possible. Reach up and place your hands on the back of your head. (If you cannot reach your head, place your arms in a "muscle man" position with elbows bent in a right angle and upper arm at shoulder level.) Take a deep breath in. As you breathe out, bring your elbows together in front of you. Slowly move elbows apart as you breathe in.

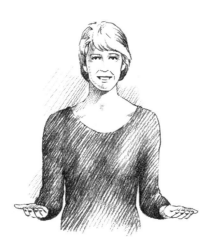
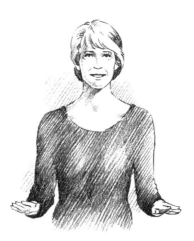

DOOR OPENER

Bend your elbows and hold them in to your sides. Your forearms should be parallel to the floor. Slowly turn forearms and palms to face the ceiling. Hold three seconds and then turn palms slowly toward the floor.

WRIST EXERCISES

Purpose: Increase wrist motion; strengthen wrist muscles.

Precautions: If you have had wrist or elbow surgery, check with your doctor before doing this exercise. Stop if you feel any numbness or tingling.

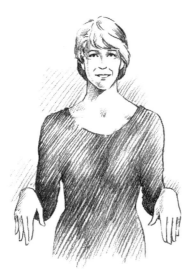
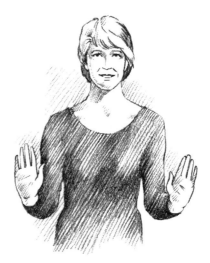

WRIST BEND (EXTENSION)

If sitting, rest hands and forearms on thighs, table, or arms of chair. If standing, bend your elbows and hold hands in front of you, palms down. Lift palms and fingers, keeping forearms flat. Hold three seconds. Relax.

FINGER EXERCISES

Purpose: Increase finger motion; increase ability to grip and hold objects.

Precautions: If the exercise increases finger pain, stop and consult with your doctor.

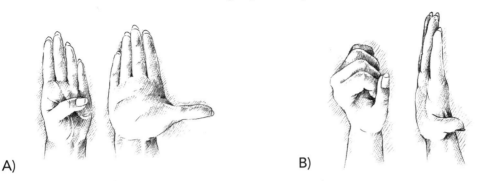

A) B)

THUMB BEND AND FINGER CURL (FLEXION/EXTENSION)

(A) With hands open and fingers relaxed, reach thumb across your palm and try to touch the base of your little finger. Hold three seconds. Stretch thumb back out to the other side as far as possible.

(B) Make a loose fist by curling all your fingers into your palm. Keep your thumb out. Hold for three seconds. Then stretch your fingers to straighten them.

TRUNK EXERCISES

Purpose: Increase trunk flexibility; stretch and strengthen back and abdominal muscles.

Precautions: If you have osteoporosis or have had back compression fracture, previous back surgery or a hip replacement, check with your doctor before doing these exercises. Do not bend your body forward or backward unless specifically told to do so. Move slowly and immediately stop any exercise that causes you back or neck pain.

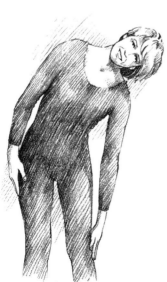

SIDE BENDS

While standing, keep weight evenly on both hips with knees slightly bent. Lean toward the right and reach your fingers toward the floor. Hold three seconds. Return to center and repeat exercise toward the left. Do not lean forward or backward while bending, and do not twist the torso.

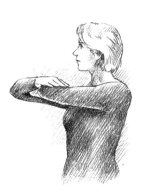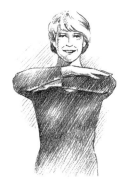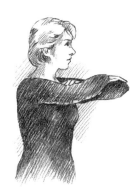

TRUNK TWIST (ROTATION)

Place your hands on your hips, straight out to the side, crossed over your chest, or on opposite elbows. Twist your body around to look over your right shoulder. Hold three seconds. Return to the center and then twist to the left. Be sure you are twisting at the waist and not at your neck or hips. NOTE: Vary the exercise by holding a ball in front of or next to your body.

LOWER-BODY EXERCISES

Purpose: Increase lower-body strength; increase range of motion in hip, knee and ankle joints. Precautions: Check with your surgeon before doing these exercises if you have had hip, knee, ankle, foot or toe surgery, or any lower-extremity joint replacement. Do not rotate the upper body unless specifically told to do so. When standing, bend your knees slightly to avoid "locking" your knee joints.

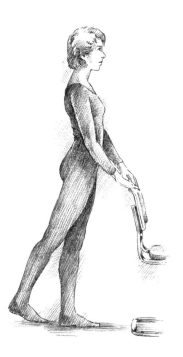

BACK KICK (HIP EXTENSION)

Stand straight on one leg and lift the other leg behind you. Hold three seconds. Try to keep your leg straight as you move it backward. Motion should occur only in the hip (not the waist). Do not lean forward – keep your upper body straight. NOTE: You can add resistance by using a large rubber exercise band around ankles.

MARCH (HIP/KNEE FLEXION)

Stand sideways to a chair and lightly grasp the back. If you feel unsteady, hold onto two chairs or face the back of the chair. Alternate lifting your legs up and down as if marching in place. Gradually try to lift knees higher and/or march faster.

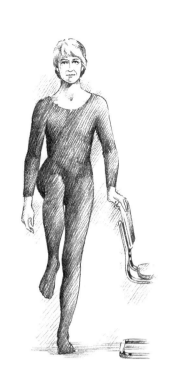

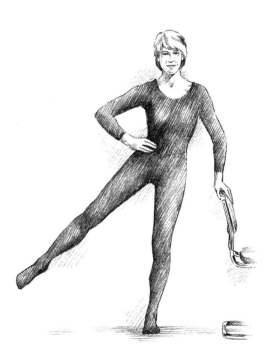

SIDE LEG KICK (HIP ABDUCTION/ADDUCTION)

Stand near a chair, holding it for support. Stand on one leg and lift the other leg out to the side. Hold three seconds and return your leg to the floor. Only move your leg at the top – don't lean toward the chair. Alternate legs.

Precautions: Check with your surgeon before doing these exercises if you have had a hip replacement. Keep the knee bent in the weight-bearing leg. Don't rotate your upper body. Keep your chest and shoulders facing forward.

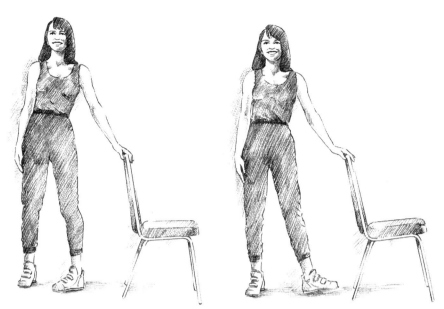

HIP TURNS (HIP INTERNAL/EXTERNAL ROTATION)

Stand with legs slightly apart, with your weight on one leg and the heel of your other foot lightly touching the floor. Rotate your whole leg from the hip so that toes and knee point in and then out. Don't rotate your body – keep chest and shoulders facing forward. NOTE: If you have difficulty putting weight on one leg, you can do this exercise by sitting at the edge of a chair with your legs extended straight in front and your heels resting on the floor.

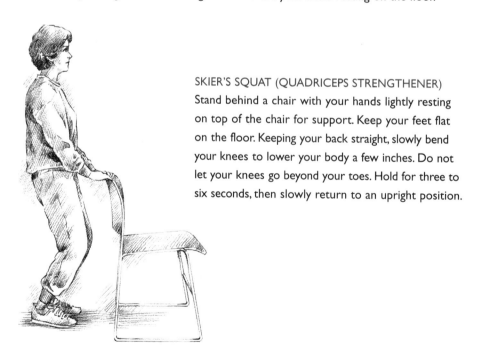

SKIER'S SQUAT (QUADRICEPS STRENGTHENER)

Stand behind a chair with your hands lightly resting on top of the chair for support. Keep your feet flat on the floor. Keeping your back straight, slowly bend your knees to lower your body a few inches. Do not let your knees go beyond your toes. Hold for three to six seconds, then slowly return to an upright position.

Precautions: Check with your surgeon before doing these exercises if you have had a hip replacement. Don't rotate your upper body. Keep your chest and shoulders facing forward.

Precautions: Do not do the following exercise if you have had ankle or foot surgery. Stop if you experience calf pain or cramping.

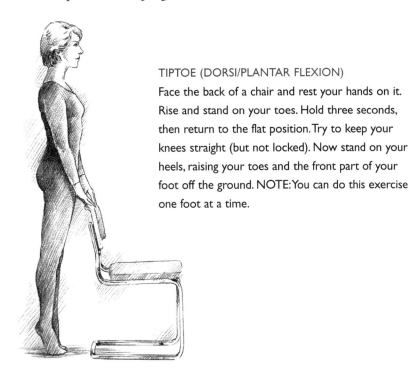

TIPTOE (DORSI/PLANTAR FLEXION)

Face the back of a chair and rest your hands on it. Rise and stand on your toes. Hold three seconds, then return to the flat position. Try to keep your knees straight (but not locked). Now stand on your heels, raising your toes and the front part of your foot off the ground. NOTE: You can do this exercise one foot at a time.

Precautions: If you have had recent ankle surgery, check with your surgeon before doing the following exercise.

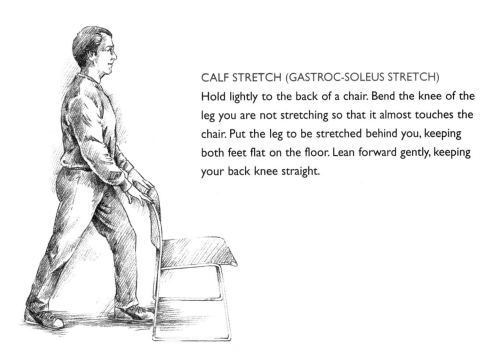

CALF STRETCH (GASTROC-SOLEUS STRETCH)

Hold lightly to the back of a chair. Bend the knee of the leg you are not stretching so that it almost touches the chair. Put the leg to be stretched behind you, keeping both feet flat on the floor. Lean forward gently, keeping your back knee straight.

Precautions: Stop if the following exercises increase your back pain.

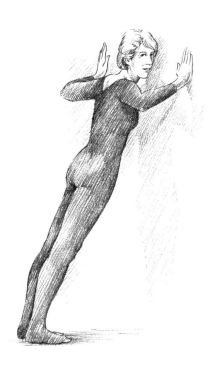

CHEST STRETCH
(HIP EXTENSION AND PECTORALIS STRETCH)

Stand about two to three feet away from a wall and place your hands or forearms on the wall at shoulder height. Lean forward, leading with your hips. Keep your knees straight and your head back. Hold this position for five to 10 seconds, then push back to starting position. To feel more stretch, place your hands farther apart.

THIGH FIRMER AND KNEE STRETCH

Sit on the edge of your chair or lie on your back with your legs stretched out in front and your heels resting on the floor. Tighten the muscle that runs across the front of the knee by pulling your toes toward your head. Push the back of the knee down toward the floor so you also feel a stretch at the back of your knee and ankle. For a greater stretch, put your heel on a footstool and lean forward as you pull your toes toward your head.

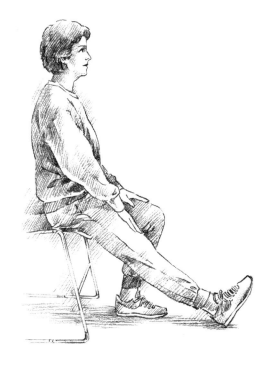

Walk Your Way to Fitness

Walking is one of the most beneficial endurance or aerobic exercises for people with fibromyalgia. Not only does walking strengthen your heart and increase your lung efficiency, it also increases your stamina and lessens your fatigue. Plus, it is inexpensive and you can do it almost anywhere.

Experts recommend that you do 30 to 40 minutes of exercise at least three times a week. For the exercise newcomer, that can seem impossible. But it doesn't have to be. Those minutes can be divided up throughout the day. The chart below provides you with a 16-week walking program that builds your endurance gradually and fits easily into the busiest of schedules.

16 Weeks to Fitness: A Walking Schedule

WEEK	Exercise Period 1 (in minutes)	Exercise Period 2 (in minutes)	Exercise Period 3 (in minutes)	Total (in minutes)
WEEK 1	2	2	2	6
WEEK 2	3	3	2	8
WEEK 3	4	3	3	10
WEEK 4	4	4	4	12
WEEK 5	5	5	5	15
WEEK 6	6	6	6	18
WEEK 7	7	7	6	20
WEEK 8	8	7	7	22
WEEK 9	8	8	8	24
WEEK 10	9	9	8	26
WEEK 11	10	9	9	28
WEEK 12	10	10	10	30
WEEK 13	11	11	10	32
WEEK 14	12	12	11	35
WEEK 15	13	13	12	38
WEEK 16	14	14	12	40

Each column represents one of the three exercise periods of each day. The schedule should be followed four days per week.

Are You Ready? A Pre-Exercise Checklist

Before you begin any new fitness program, be sure you are prepared. The following checklist can help:

❑ **Have you consulted with your physician or physical therapist?** Always talk to your health-care team before beginning any new fitness program.

❑ **Are you wearing comfortable clothes?** Clothes should be loose and worn in layers. Breathable, easily washable fabrics are best.

❑ **Are your shoes right for you?** Ill-fitting or inappropriate shoes can cause a world of ache on your feet. Make sure your shoes provide support for your arches and have non-slip, shock-absorbent insoles.

❑ **Have you warmed up properly?** A warm-up period not only gets you mentally charged to start your aerobic exercise, it also gets your body ready to start its workout and helps prevent injuries. (For sample warm-up exercises, see pages 75–84.)

The Talk Test

Are you exercising at an appropriate level during your aerobic activity? To find out, take the talk test. If you cannot carry on a conversation while exercising without feeling out of breath, then you are pushing it too hard. Slow down a bit until you are working at a comfortable level.

Water Exercise

Water exercise, especially in warm water, is great for stiff, sore muscles. It also helps support your body by putting less stress on your hips, knees and spine.

Water exercise is not limited to swimming only. There are many warm-water exercises you can do while standing in shoulder- or chest-high water. The following warm-water exercise examples have been excerpted from the Arthritis Foundation's patient education booklet *Water Exercise: Pools, Spas and Arthritis.* To order a free copy, call 800/283-7800 or log on to www.arthritis.org. To find a warm-water exercise program near you, contact your local Arthritis Foundation chapter.

HIPS AND KNEES

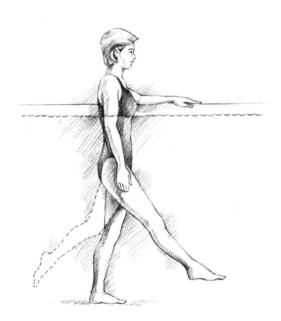

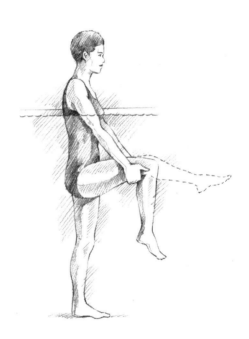

LEG SWING (HIP FLEXION/EXTENSION)

- Stand with one side against the pool wall, and hold on for balance.
- Perform slowly.
- Bring your thigh parallel to the water surface as high as is comfortable.
- Lower your leg.
- Gently swing your leg behind you.
- Repeat with other side.

KNEE LIFT (HIP AND KNEE FLEXION/EXTENSION)

- Stand with one side against the pool wall.
- Bend your knee, bringing your thigh parallel to the water's surface as high as is comfortable.
- Cup one hand behind your knee if your leg needs extra support.
- Straighten your knee and then lower your leg, keeping the knee straight.
- Keep your ankles and toes relaxed.
- Repeat on the other side.

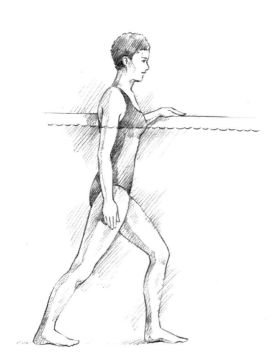

CALF STRETCH

- Stand with your side toward the wall, and place your hand on the wall for balance.
- Stand straight with your legs slightly apart and with one leg ahead of the other.
- Keep your body straight, lean forward and slowly let your front knee bend. You will feel the stretch on the calf of your back leg. Your heel on the back leg should stay on the floor.
- Hold the stretch for 10 seconds.
- Repeat with your other leg.

SIDE LEG LIFT
(HIP ABDUCTION AND ADDUCTION)

- Stand with your side to the pool wall, with your knees relaxed. Place your hand on the wall for balance.
- Swing your leg out to the side, toward the center of the pool and in toward the wall, crossing in front of your other leg. Repeat on the other side.

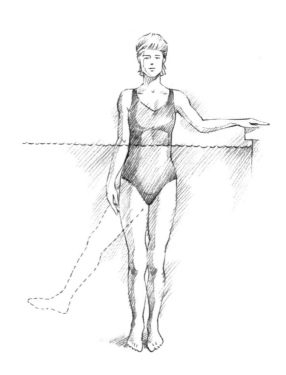

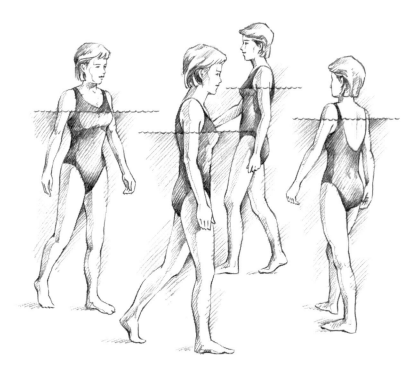

WALKING

- Walk normally across or in a circle in the pool. Swing your arms as you walk.
- Wearing water shoes or sneakers is helpful.

TRUNK

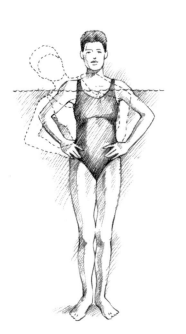

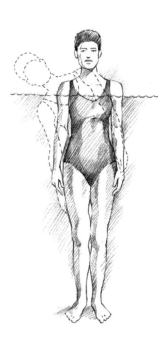

SIDE BEND (FLEXION)

- Place your hands on your hips with your feet shoulder-width apart and knees relaxed.
- Bend slowly to one side, with your hand sliding down your thigh as you bend.
- Return to starting position and bend to other side. Do not bend forward or twist or turn your trunk.

SHOULDERS

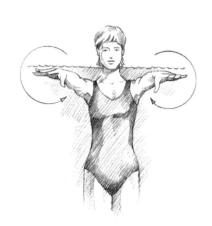

ARM CIRCLES
- Raise both arms in front of you until they are a few inches below water level.
- Keep both elbows straight. Make small circles (about the size of a softball) with your arms.
- Gradually increase the circles' size (until they are the size of a basketball), and then decrease them to the size of softballs again.
- First make clockwise circles, then counterclockwise circles. Do not raise your arms out of the water or let them cross.

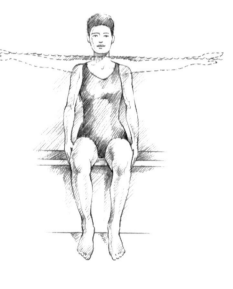

SIDEWAYS ARM REACH (ABDUCTION)
- Slowly raise both arms out to the side, keeping your palms down. Raise only to shoulder (water) level.
- Lower your arms. Do not shrug your shoulders or twist your trunk.

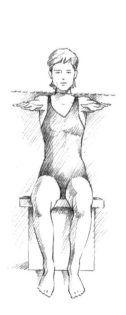
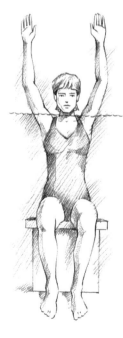

FORWARD ARM REACH (FLEXION)
- With both arms, reach straight in front of you.
- Raise your hands overhead as high as possible, keeping your elbows as straight as you can.

ELBOWS

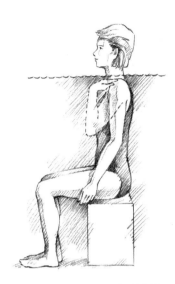

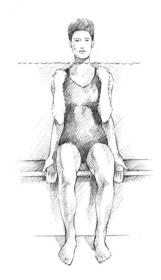

ELBOW BEND (FLEXION/EXTENSION)

- Bend your elbows, bringing your thumbs toward your shoulders.
- Straighten your arms at your sides.

ELBOW BEND AND TURN

- Turn your arms until the palms face forward.
- Bend the elbows until your fingertips touch your shoulders.
- Keep your palms up when raising your hands; the backs of your hands push the water down.
- Keep your elbows close to your body.

HANDS AND FINGERS

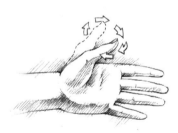

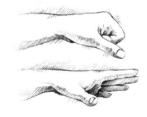

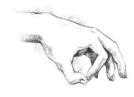

THUMB CIRCLES (CIRCUMDUCTION)

- Move your thumb in large circles.
- Then reverse directions.

FINGER CURL (FLEXION/EXTENSION)

- Bend each joint slowly to make a loose fist.
- Then straighten them out.

FINGER HOLD (THUMB OPPOSITION)

- Touch the tip of your left thumb to the tips of your other fingers on that hand, one at a time, to form a round "O."
- Open hand wide after each "O."

WRISTS AND FINGERS

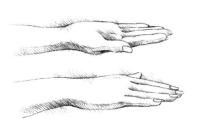

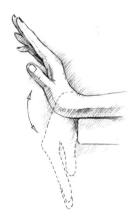

WRIST TURN (SUPINATION/PRONATION)

- Turn your palms toward the ceiling.
- Turn them down to face the bottom of the hot tub or pool. Keep your elbows near your waist.

WRIST BEND (FLEXION/EXTENSION)

- Bend both wrists upward and then downward. Hands and fingers should be relaxed.

ANKLES AND TOES

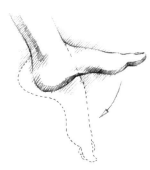

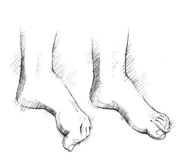

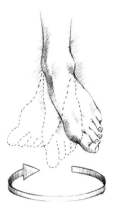

ANKLE BEND (DORSIFLEXION/PLANTAR FLEXION)

- Place your weight on one foot and hold to the side of the pool for support.
- Bend your foot up, then down. Repeat with your other foot.

TOE CURL (FLEXION/EXTENSION)

- Place your weight on one foot and hold to the side of the pool for support.
- Lift your knee slightly. Curl your toes down, then straighten them out.
- Repeat with your other foot.

ANKLE CIRCLES (DORSIFLEXION/PLANTAR FLEXION AND INVERSION/EVERSION)

- Place your weight on one foot and hold to the side of the pool for support.
- Make large inward circles, moving it at the ankle.
- Repeat circles in the opposite direction, then repeat the exercise with your other foot.

HIPS AND KNEES

KNEE BEND (FLEXION/EXTENSION)

- Sit on the edge of the seat.
- Bend knee, putting heel back as far as possible.
- Bring foot up, straightening knee out slowly.
- Repeat with other leg.

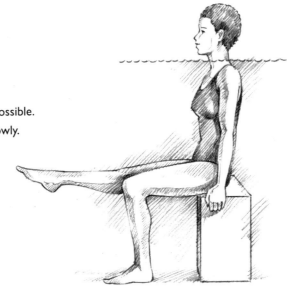

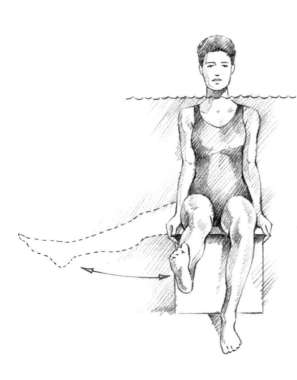

SPREAD EAGLE
(HIP ABDUCTION WITH KNEE EXTENSION)

- Sit on the edge of the seat and straighten one knee.
- While holding it straight, slowly move it out to the side.
- Bring it back to the center and relax.
- Repeat with your other leg.

Ai Chi: Peace in the Water

It's a paradox people with fibromyalgia know all too well: Avoiding pain has meant avoiding excessive movement, particularly exercise. But the way to move out of a deconditioned state and build back strength – and eventually lessen pain – is to exercise.

An activity that seems tailor-made to deal with the fibromyalgia exercise Catch-22 is Ai Chi, which has grown in popularity around the United States since its development in Japan in the mid-1990s. Ai Chi evolved from Watsu, a high-touch form of warm-water body work based on shiatsu massage that is used in both therapeutic and non-therapeutic settings.

Performed in chest-deep warm water (between 86 and 92 degrees Fahrenheit), either alone or with a group, Ai Chi is a combination exercise/meditation technique that combines deep breathing with slow, broad movements of the arms, legs and torso. The pain-relieving and buoyancy properties of the warm water allow those with fibromyalgia to practice in a pain-free fashion a variety of range-of-motion and strengthening techniques they might be unable to do on land. And, says one Ai Chi aficionado with fibromyalgia, there is no "morning-after" exercise hangover after a typical 45-minute Ai Chi session.

However, Ai Chi may not be for everyone. People with unstable blood pressure, open wounds, sensitivity to pool chemicals and certain other medical conditions should not engage in Ai Chi. It also may not be appropriate for people who are afraid of the water, although it is not necessary to know how to swim in order to participate. Remember, as with any exercise program, consult with a doctor before beginning a new regimen.

To find out where Ai Chi is being taught near you, contact local YWCAs and YMCAs, community pools and health clubs.

Find Your Target Heart Rate

Your target heart rate refers to the level of physical exertion that you aim for in your exercise routine. As you exercise, your heart rate should increase to a higher level than it is when you are sitting still. It's important to achieve a certain target heart rate as you

exercise so your workout is successful.

To find your target heart rate, you must stop during your activity and take your pulse. Keep walking or moving around to keep your blood circulating. Placing your index and middle fingers on your opposite wrist or below your jawline on your neck, count your pulse for six seconds and add a zero to that number (or count for 10 seconds and multiply by six). For example, if you count 14 beats in a 10-second period, your heart rate is six times 14, or 84 beats per minute.

Using the chart for a guide, find the target heart rate for your age group. You don't want your heart rate to be faster than the top end of the range during your aerobic exercise. If it does exceed the maximum, slow it down! If you are a beginner, consider the higher number in your range as a "not-to-exceed" heart rate. And take heart: if you exercise in your target range regularly, your endurance and conditioning will improve.

Recommended Heart Rate Ranges

AGE	HEART RATE RANGE (60%-75% of Age-Predicted Maximum Heart Rate)	10-SECOND COUNT
20	120 – 150	20 – 25
25	117 – 146	19 – 24
30	114 – 143	19 – 24
35	111 – 139	18 – 23
40	108 – 135	18 – 23
45	105 – 131	17 – 22
50	102 – 128	17 – 21
55	99 – 124	16 – 21
60	96 – 120	16 – 20
65	93 – 116	15 – 19
70	90 – 113	15 – 19
75	87 – 109	14 – 18
80	84 – 105	14 – 18
85	81 – 101	13 – 17
90	78 – 98	13 – 16

Put It in Writing

It's easy to forget the promises you make to yourself about starting a fitness program or sticking to it. If you really want to keep your promise, put it in writing. Make copies of the chart on the opposite page and post it on your refrigerator to record your daily activity.

Keeping an exercise diary will not only remind you to stick to your fitness program, it will show you the progress you've made. A sample is shown below.

Exercise Diary Sample

Photocopy this chart and use it to keep records of your exercise activities.

Date/Time	Exercises	Frequency/ Duration	Heart Rate	Feelings/ Comments
8/10	Walk	30 min.	121	great! pumped up
8/12	Yoga	50 min.	108	Sore but relaxed
8/16	Walk	45 min.	125	stiff – need to keep active
8/17	Walk	30 min.	120	better – keep it up!

ACTIVITY

Exercise Diary

Photocopy this chart and use it to keep records of your exercise activities.

Date/Time	Exercises	Frequency/ Duration	Heart Rate	Feelings/ Comments

GOOD LIVING
GOOD LIVING
GOOD LIVING
GOOD LIVING
GOOD LIVING
GOOD LIVING
GOOD LIVING
GOOD LIVING
GOOD LIVING

CHAPTER 7:

Eating Well

Eating well won't cure your fibromyalgia, but it will make you feel better. Eating a balanced diet will help your body function at its very best. Learn to incorporate more fruits and vegetables into your diet, cut out added sugar and caffeine, and see how quickly you begin to feel stronger, healthier and more energetic.

Are You Eating Wisely?

Research has not shown that any specific foods affect fibromyalgia, but it has been proven that a balanced diet can help you feel better and stay healthy. Balancing your diet does not mean you have to eliminate the foods you love. Instead, stick to the Food Guide Pyramid (*see below*) and follow these suggestions:

- Include fiber, fruits, vegetables and calcium-rich foods in your diet.

- Reduce the amount of salt, fat, cholesterol and sugar you consume.

- Limit your alcohol and caffeine intake.

- Drink eight to 12 (8 oz.) glasses of water every day.

- Eat three to five servings of vegetables and two to three servings of fruits every day.

The Food Guide Pyramid

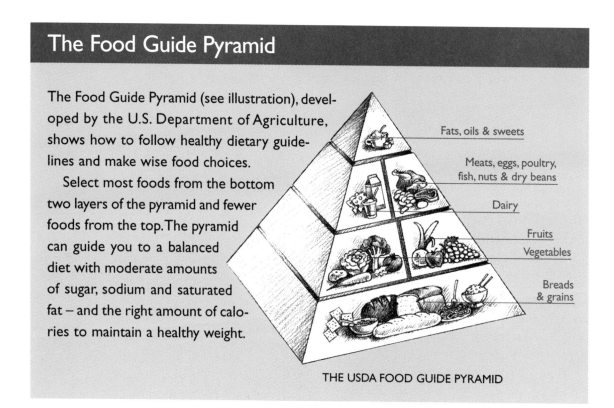

The Food Guide Pyramid (see illustration), developed by the U.S. Department of Agriculture, shows how to follow healthy dietary guidelines and make wise food choices.

Select most foods from the bottom two layers of the pyramid and fewer foods from the top. The pyramid can guide you to a balanced diet with moderate amounts of sugar, sodium and saturated fat – and the right amount of calories to maintain a healthy weight.

Fats, oils & sweets

Meats, eggs, poultry, fish, nuts & dry beans

Dairy

Fruits

Vegetables

Breads & grains

THE USDA FOOD GUIDE PYRAMID

Diet "Cures": Are They For Real?

You may read about special diets or a supplements that claim to cure health problems. But most of them are unproven, and many of them are just rip-offs. Use this checklist to determine if the latest "cure" is a fraud:

❏ It advises you to eliminate an essential food group from the Food Guide Pyramid.

❏ It stresses that you eat only a few foods or eliminate certain foods.

❏ It claims to cure fibromyalgia.

❏ It uses misleading advertisements that look like news articles.

❏ It lacks scientific evidence, such as published studies, to back its claims.

❏ It promotes a diet that you suspect could be harmful to your health.

Food Diary

The best way to evaluate your diet to see if you are eating sensibly is to write down what you eat in a food diary. If you are concerned about weight gain, you can share your food diary with your doctor or a dietitian who can help you develop a healthy diet. You can lose weight without starving yourself of the foods you love and the nutrients you need.

Food Diary Sample

Breakfast

Cereal w/ milk   Water (w/ pills)
Banana   Orange juice

Lunch

Turkey sandwich w/ lettuce and mayo (light)

Food Diary

Photocopy this chart and use it to record your daily dietary intake.

Breakfast

Lunch

Dinner

Snack

Water (8 to 12 glasses per day) ❑ ❑ ❑ ❑ ❑ ❑ ❑ ❑ ❑ ❑ ❑ ❑

Fruits (at least 2 to 5 servings per day) ❑ ❑ ❑ ❑ ❑

Vegetables (at least 3 to 5 servings per day) ❑ ❑ ❑ ❑ ❑

Make Meal Preparation Easy

Sometimes the pain or fatigue of fibromyalgia can keep you from doing even the most basic tasks, like making dinner. Answer the questions below to see if you are doing all you can to make meal preparation easier on yourself:

❑ YES ❑ NO

Do you plan rest breaks during meal preparation?

❑ YES ❑ NO

Do you use good posture to avoid pain during cooking tasks?

❑ YES ❑ NO

Have you arranged your kitchen for convenience? Do you keep the tools you use most within easy reach?

❑ YES ❑ NO

Do you buy healthy convenience food, such as sliced and chopped vegetables?

❑ YES ❑ NO

Do you add fresh fruit and bread to a frozen dinner for a simple, satisfying meal?

❑ YES ❑ NO

Do you use kitchen appliances and tools, such as electric can openers and microwave ovens, that save you time and effort?

❑ YES ❑ NO

When you share meals with friends or family members, do you split the cooking tasks and enjoy the company?

GOOD LIVING
GOOD LIVING
GOOD LIVING
GOOD LIVING
GOOD LIVING
GOOD LIVING
GOOD LIVING
GOOD LIVING
GOOD LIVING
GOOD LIVING

CHAPTER 8:

Getting Along

While your body bears the brunt of the effects of fibromyalgia, your relationships with others also are affected. Your personal relationships can become strained under the weight of your condition.

Keeping the lines of communication open is your best step toward getting the support you need from your loved ones. And building a support network of family and friends, to rely on during trying moments is vital to the management of your condition.

How Well Do You Communicate?

Sometimes it's difficult for the people in your life to understand how fibromyalgia makes you feel. If you can't communicate your feelings effectively, how can you get the support you need? Use the questionnaire below to see if you are doing all that you can to communicate your feelings effectively.

❏ YES ❏ NO Do you use "I" messages? Instead of putting the other person on the defensive by using "you" statements (e.g., "You make me angry when you do that."), "I" messages are factual statements about how you feel that do not place blame on the other person (e.g., "I am angry that you did that.").

❏ YES ❏ NO Do you listen? Being a good listener is essential to good communication. Be sure to show that you are lis-tening by using nonverbal and verbal cues that show you are interested, such as a nod or an encouraging, "Go on."

❏ YES ❏ NO Do you ask for more information? If you don't clearly understand what someone else is com-municating, it is up to you to get the information you need to understand. Ask for more information or ask about the meaning of what was said. Be spe-cific in your questions.

❏ YES ❏ NO Do you educate others? When the miscommunication involves your fibromyalgia, it's usually because the other person doesn't understand your condition. Become a fibromyalgia advo-cate and help others understand what fibromyalgia is all about.

Guide to Intimacy

To learn new approaches to sex when you have a chronic illness, such as fibromyalgia, contact the Arthritis Foundation for a copy of the free *Arthritis Today* reprint, "The Arthritis Foundation's Guide to Intimacy and Arthritis." Call 800/283-7800 for more information or visit www.arthritis.org.

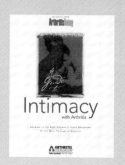

ACTIVITY

Let's Talk About Sex

Fibromyalgia can affect your sexuality in several ways, both physical and emotional. However, you may be nervous to talk about sex with your partner, not knowing where to begin. Use the worksheet below to write out your feelings and thoughts about sex and share them with your partner.

Has fibromyalgia altered your sexual relationship or your feelings about sex? _____

_____

What, if anything, has changed? _____

_____

What is more or less the same? _____

_____

Are there any sexual activities that are not as pleasant as they used to be? _____

_____

Are there any that are more enjoyable? _____

_____

Does lovemaking cause any particular problems for you or your partner? _____

_____

Where on your body do you enjoy being touched? Where is touching unpleasant? _____

_____

Are there new things you would like to try? If so, what are they? _____

_____

Have you talked to your partner about any of these things? _____

_____

Problem-Solving

Despite your best efforts, sometimes communication fails. Don't give up. Instead, write your feelings down. Putting your problem down on paper may be the quickest way to develop a solution. Photocopy this worksheet and use it to help.

1. Select a current problem or concern and list any known causes.
2. Write down several possible solutions for dealing with this problem or its causes.
3. Consider the advantages and disadvantages of each option.
4. Select an option to try.
5. Evaluate your results after implementing the option selected.

1. Problem/Cause

2. Possible Solutions

3. Advantages   **Disadvantages**

4. Option to Try

5. Results/Outcome

Build a Support Network

Sometimes you have to go outside of your close-knit network of family and friends to get the support you need. Many people with fibromyalgia find encouragement from support groups. People in support groups can share their feelings about their condition and learn from one another.

To find a fibromyalgia support group near you, contact one of the following groups listed below:

- The Arthritis Foundation can help you find a support group in your area. Call your local chapter or find a chapter near you by calling 800/283-7800 or visiting www.arthritis.org.

- The National Fibromyalgia Partnership publishes the 154-page *North American Directory of Fibromyalgia Support Services*, which includes a comprehensive listing of active groups in the U.S., Canada and Mexico, with details on the types of programs that the group provides, any fees involved, etc. The directory costs $25 for members, $38 for others. The organization also provides listings for specific states, which are free by e-mail or cost $1 by mail (send a business SASE). Contact the association at 140 Zinn Way, Linden, VA 22642-5609; e-mail to mail@fmpartnership.org; or visit their Web site at www.fmpartnership.org.

- The National Fibromyalgia Association maintains a list of support groups and other resources that can help you. E-mail nfa@fmaware.org; or visit their Web site at www.fmaware.org.

What a Support Group Can Do For You

Support groups can offer a variety of programs to help members develop their own support systems. Check off the benefits that you think could help you:

- ❏ Details of upcoming events, such as health fairs, conferences and workshops
- ❏ Programs on alternative therapies, such as massage, yoga or water therapy
- ❏ Information, shared among the participants, on particularly helpful and well-informed health care providers
- ❏ Tips on daily living issues, such as finding a grocery store where employees are helpful with your particular needs
- ❏ Programs for the families and loved ones of group members to discuss their logistical and emotional challenges
- ❏ Presentations by various experts, including doctors, therapists and other professionals, on such topics as diet and exercise, and details and impact of current research findings

Talking to Your Boss

Fibromyalgia affects every aspect of your life, from your physical abilities to your relationships with others. Your workplace is no exception. If you are experiencing cognitive or concentration problems or having problems performing strenuous tasks you were once able to do, then maybe it's time to talk to your employer about your condition.

The following tips may help:

- **Be prepared.** Plan what you are going to say ahead of time. Equip yourself with resources, such as articles and brochures. Give your supervisor a copy of the Fibromyalgia patient education booklet from the Arthritis Foundation (call 800/283-7800 to receive a free copy). Be prepared to discuss different options for making your work environment more fibro-friendly.

- **Be honest.** Employers can't help unless they know what is wrong. Explain your work needs and the specifics of your condition.

- **Be positive.** Stress the things you can do, focusing on your experience, education and enthusiasm. Explain how special equipment and/or special accommodations would help you do your job better and more productively.

- **Be creative.** Think up different ways your working conditions can be adapted to help you cope with your fibromyalgia and be a productive employee. Just because it hasn't been done before doesn't mean it can't be done. If you're too tired at the end of the day to get the much-needed exercise to help your fibromyalgia, ask if you can have two hours for lunch and work an hour later, so you can eat and go to the gym during lunch. Or ask if you can move your office to the first floor so you don't have to climb stairs every day.

GOOD LIVING
GOOD LIVING
GOOD LIVING
GOOD LIVING
GOOD LIVING
GOOD LIVING
GOOD LIVING
GOOD LIVING
GOOD LIVING

GOOD LIVING
GOOD LIVING
GOOD LIVING
GOOD LIVING
GOOD LIVING
GOOD LIVING
GOOD LIVING
GOOD LIVING
GOOD LIVING

CHAPTER 9:

In Control

Fibromyalgia may have changed your life in innumerable ways, but that doesn't mean you have to let it rule your life. Nor should you let other people dictate how you manage your condition.

Be proactive in your treatment plan. Learn all you can about fibromyalgia and take part in making decisions that affect your health. The activities in this chapter will help you set goals for yourself and take charge of your fibromyalgia.

Are You a Self-Manager?

Being a self-manager means that you take charge of your fibromyalgia *and* your life. Do you have what it takes to be a successful self-manager? Test yourself:

❏ **Are you learning all you can about fibromyalgia?** Understanding your condition will make you feel less helpless. Talk to health-care professionals, support groups and other people with fibromyalgia. Read about it in books, newspapers and on the Internet. Contact your local chapter of the Arthritis Foundation.

❏ **Are you an active member of your health-care team?** Don't rely on your health-care providers alone to treat your fibromyalgia. To get the most out of your treatment, you need to be actively involved in the decision-making about your health. Talk to your doctor about your symptoms, side effects and feelings. Write down questions and concerns. Monitor your progress and report any

changes. The worksheets in this workbook can help you.

❏ **Are you leading a healthy lifestyle?** In order to "feel" healthy, you have to be healthy. That means exercising regularly, eating a balanced diet, getting plenty of rest and doing things that make you happy.

❏ **Are you taking responsibility for the things you can control?** Only you can control your thoughts and actions. Commit yourself to doing everything you can to make yourself feel better by setting goals for yourself, getting help when you need it and learning to accept the things you can't control.

❏ **Are you the master of your emotional well-being?** Be open about your feelings and frustrations. Learn stress-reduction and relaxation exercises that will better help you deal with the day-to-day stresses of living with fibromyalgia. Get help if you need it.

ACTIVITY

Contract for a Better Life With Fibromyalgia

Setting goals for yourself – and sticking to them – is an essential part of being a self-manager. One way to make sure you follow through with your goals is to make a contract with yourself. Photocopy the form on the following page, and use it to make a contract with yourself to accomplish one of your weekly goals.

Contract Form

THIS WEEK I WILL: _____ WEEK OF: _____

For Example: This week I will <u>walk</u> <u>around the block</u> <u>before lunch</u> <u>three times.</u>
                              (WHAT)   (HOW MUCH)   (WHEN)   (HOW MANY)

What

How Much

When

How Many Days

How Certain Are You
(On a scale of 0 to 10 with 0 being totally unsure and 10 being totally confident)

Signature

THIS WEEK I WILL: _____ WEEK OF: _____

What

How Much

When

How Many Days

How Certain Are You
(On a scale of 0 to 10 with 0 being totally unsure and 10 being totally confident)

Signature

Put It in Writing

Because fibromyalgia varies from person to person, many doctors rely on their patients to keep track of symptoms, pains and feelings associated with their fibromyalgia. Doctors can use this information to identify patterns and inconsistencies and to develop better treatment plans for their patients.

For you, recording your experiences provides you with concrete documentation of your symptoms and helps you communicate with your medical team as well as family and friends.

There are many ways to record your experiences with fibromyalgia. This workbook abounds with examples, including diaries for food (page 102) and exercise (page 97), sleep (page 139) and stress (page 150). The following pages offer more diary examples, such as a mood and pain diary and an activities diary. Use them together to help plan your more strenuous activities for when you are feeling at your best.

Writing for You

While many of the diaries in this workbook are intended to be shared with your healthcare team or members of your support network, you may also want to consider keeping one just for yourself.

Many people with fibromyalgia have found that keeping a diary or journal helps them come to terms with their feelings

about their condition. Journaling provides you with a forum to open up about your thoughts and frustrations and everyday ups and downs. Journaling also allows you to be honest without having to worry about sparing another person's feelings or about how others perceive you.

Get Started: Pick Up a Pen

Here are some journaling pointers to get you started:

- Keep a journal handy at all times. Carry one with you and keep one in the car.
- Set a specific time to journal daily, whether it's at 11 a.m. or just before bedtime.
- Don't worry about guidelines as to how much you should write. Follow your instincts.
- Write strictly for yourself (even if you eventually share it with others). Don't get hung up on grammar, punctuation or technique.

ACTIVITY

Mood and Pain Diary

It is useful to monitor your pain level and mood to learn more about possible associations. Photocopy this chart and use it to rate your current mood and pain level on the 0-10 scale. For the next week, rate your pain and mood three times per day (e.g., a.m. — when you get up in the morning, midday and p.m. — before going to bed). Then look for patterns or possible associations.

FOR EACH TIME PERIOD

- Mark an **X** across from the number that describes your **mood**; (0 = best mood, 10 = worst mood or most anxious/depressed/negative feelings).

MOOD/PAIN DIARY

	a.m.	Mid-Day	p.m.	a.m.	Mid-Day	p.m.	a.m.	Mid-Day	p.m.	a.m.	Mid-Day	p.m.	a.m.	Mid-Day	p.m.	a.m.	Mid-Day	p.m.	a.m.	Mid-Day	p.m.
10																					
9																					
8																					
7																					
6																					
5																					
4																					
3																					
2																					
1																					
0																					
	Mon/Day 1			Tue/Day 2			Wed/Day 3			Thur/Day 4			Fri/Day 5			Sat/Day 6			Sun/Day 7		

ACTIVITY

Activities Diary

Photocopy this worksheet and use it to help you analyze how you spend a typical week. Record what you are doing at that time (e.g., 7 a.m. — Breakfast). Then compare it with the Mood and Pain diary to determine when you are at your best, and you can adjust your activities accordingly.

	MON	TUE	WED	THUR	FRI	SAT	SUN
6 a.m.							
7 a.m.							
8 a.m.							
9 a.m.							
10 a.m.							
11 a.m.							
noon							
1 p.m.							
2 p.m.							
3 p.m.							
4 p.m.							
5 p.m.							
6 p.m.							
7 p.m.							
8 p.m.							
9 p.m.							
10 p.m.							
11 p.m.							
midnight							

GOOD LIVING
GOOD LIVING
GOOD LIVING
GOOD LIVING
GOOD LIVING
GOOD LIVING
GOOD LIVING
GOOD LIVING
GOOD LIVING

GOOD LIVING
GOOD LIVING
GOOD LIVING
GOOD LIVING
GOOD LIVING
GOOD LIVING
GOOD LIVING
GOOD LIVING
GOOD LIVING

CHAPTER 10:

Closing the Gates

Whether it's sharp, stabbing pains or an all-over ache, pain is a constant reminder that you have fibromyalgia. And until there is a miraculous medicine that will make your fibromyalgia pain go away, you have to rely on a variety of pain-management techniques. Some people prefer such treatments as massage or biofeedback, while others rely on mind-body exercises.

The activities in this chapter offer a sampling of pain-management strategies you can use to take control of your fibromyalgia pain.

How Do You Manage Your Pain?

Chapter 10 of the *Arthritis Foundation's Guide to Good Living with Fibromyalgia* discusses how pain works and details methods you can use to manage it. Which methods do you use to close the gates on pain?

❑ Heat and cold treatments. These treatments are easy ways to reduce pain by relaxing your muscles and stimulating circulation.

❑ Exercise. A gentle exercise program will increase your flexibility and relieve stiffness as well as give you an improved sense of well-being.

❑ Massage. Massage temporarily relieves pain, muscle tension and spasms by increasing blood flow and warming sore areas.

❑ Mind-body techniques. Treatments like yoga and biofeedback help reduce your body's stress response and improve the delivery of oxygen to your muscles and brain.

❑ Relaxation. Practicing relaxation exercises can help you relax your muscles and lower your heart rate and blood pressure during stressful times.

❑ Distraction. Simply taking your mind off your pain by focusing on something else can help you become less aware of your discomfort.

❑ Humor. Laughter not only is a great distraction from your pain, it also is beneficial to your health, staving off pain by producing endorphins.

Straighten Up: Posture Tips

Proper posture will not cure fibromyalgia, but it may ease your pain and strengthen weak or damaged muscles. Good upright posture eases stress on the muscles and ligaments and also corrects muscle imbalances that lead to pain.

To achieve good posture, it's important to remind yourself to stand and sit correctly throughout the day. Every morning or evening, do a few exercises that keep your back aligned. Pretty soon good posture will become more automatic.

Here are some pointers to help you maintain correct back posture:

SITTING:

- Try to take breaks from sitting every hour, and more often if you're in pain.
- Make sure your back is supported by a chair with a firm seat and back.
- Sit with your knees slightly higher than your hips to keep your back from arching.
- Don't cross your legs; do sit with feet firmly planted on the ground.
- If your chair doesn't adjust so your feet touch the ground, or if you can't maintain good posture, you may need a stool for your feet.

continued on page 124

Exercises To Improve Your Posture

The following exercises can help strengthen your muscles and improve your posture. If you experience radiating pain or numbness during these exercises, you should consult your doctor.

SCAPULAR PINCH

- Lift your hands to the shoulder level with elbows bent.
- Keep your elbows pointing down and pinch your shoulders back.
- Hold the position briefly for about two breaths.
- Repeat three times.

BACK EXTENSION

- Place your palms on your lower back while standing or sitting.
- Gently lean backward in a stretch.
- Hold the position briefly for about two breaths.
- Repeat three times.

HIP STRETCH

- Hold onto your lower leg, just below the knee, while sitting.
- Gently pull the leg towards your chest, allowing the knee to bend.
- Hold the position for about two breaths.
- Repeat three times.

ABDOMINAL STRENGTHENING

- Lie down on a mat or rug, or against several pillows in a sit-up position. Have someone hold your feet or tuck them under a piece of furniture.
- As you sit up, hold your lower stomach in and hold your breath, keeping your back in a C-curve, pressing the small of your back down.
- As you come back down to a lying position, breathe out. Do the exercise smoothly, without jerks or starts.
- Repeat five times.

continued from page 122

STANDING:

- Stand straight with the shoulders and head held up and back. Imagine a string in the center of your head pulling upwards. By tightening your abdominal muscles, you can also support your spine.
- If you have to stand for more than 10 minutes, place one foot on a low stool to relieve pressure on your spine, and change positions every 10 or 15 minutes (or more often if needed).
- Don't wear high-heeled shoes or boots, which tend to cause you to have a "sway" back (an overly arched back).

- If you stand while performing your job, stand on a padded surface or place padding in your shoes. Try to stand with weight evenly distributed on both feet.

SLEEPING:

- Unless you already have one, get a good firm mattress.
- If you sleep on your back, try elevating your legs on pillows for relief of pain. A neck pillow may also help.
- Place a pillow between your legs if you sleep on your side.
- For face-down sleeping, place a pillow under your stomach and feet.

Think Your Pain Away

The healing power of positive thinking is not just bunk invented by self-help gurus. It's scientifically proven, and there are therapists who can help you battle the pain of fibromyalgia with a little cognitive behavioral therapy.

Cognitive behavioral therapy (CBT) is a treatment that helps people identify thoughts that promote disabling behavior, develop strategies to change those thoughts and devise new approaches.

Developed by psychiatrist Aaron Beck in the 1960s, CBT typically requires weekly meetings with a therapist who helps patients see that distorted beliefs are limiting their capabilities. Are you prone to distorted beliefs? Some examples of distorted thinking include:

- Polarized or all-or-nothing thinking – seeing every situation as black or white.
- Mental filtering – focusing on negative elements, ignoring any positives.
- Overgeneralization – predicting negative outcomes based on one bad experience.
- Personalizing – blaming yourself for negative outcomes even when circumstances are beyond your control.
- Mind reading – assuming that others are thinking negatively of you.

To break distorted thinking patterns, therapists use worksheets and activities like the ones in this workbook to help people with fibromyalgia change the way they think about their condition and the negative effects it has had on their lives.

ACTIVITY

Create Your Own Pain-Management Plan

How do you plan on controlling your pain? Use these worksheets to chart your pain-management plan. Make copies of them and post them where you can refer to them often.

MY PAIN-MANAGEMENT PLAN

Use the following worksheet to record the strategies you plan to use for pain relief. That way you'll have a ready reference when you need it.

Medications:

_____

_____

Schedule:

_____

_____

Heat, cold, massage:

_____

_____

Relaxation techniques:

_____

_____

Exercises:

_____

_____

Other techniques (distraction, humor, pleasant thoughts):

_____

_____

continued page 126

Pain-Management Plan (continued)

I take these medications at these times: _____

Name of medication: _____

Schedule: _____

Heat, cold or massage can help my pain. What I will do: _____

_____

When I will do it: _____

_____

Rest is important in managing my pain. I will rest: _____

_____

Exercise can help my pain and stiffness. I will do (types of exercises): _____

_____

I will do these exercises (how often/when): _____

_____

Being calm and relaxed helps the pain. My ways to practice relaxation are: _____

_____

I will practice these techniques _____ times a day.

Keeping my mind off the pain is important. When I'm in pain, I will think about (list some pleasant

thoughts or memories): _____

_____

I need to focus on healthful habits. One new healthful habit I'm going to practice is:

_____

I'm going to ask my doctor or therapist these questions about my treatment program:

_____

Resources, addresses & phone numbers: _____

Local Arthritis Foundation chapter: _____

Local fibromyalgia organization: _____

Doctor: _____

Therapist(s): _____

Pharmacist: _____

Other members of my health-care team: _____

_____

GOOD LIVING
GOOD LIVING
GOOD LIVING
GOOD LIVING
GOOD LIVING
GOOD LIVING
GOOD LIVING
GOOD LIVING
GOOD LIVING

CHAPTER 11:

Feeling Exhausted

Feeling run-down most of the time? You probably are experiencing fatigue, like 75 percent to 80 percent of the fibromyalgia population. There are steps you can take, however, to keep fatigue from preventing you from doing the things you love to do.

Priority-setting and time management may help you find your balance between doing too much and succumbing to exhaustion. The activities in this chapter will help you learn to cope with fatigue.

Set Your Priorities Straight

For many people with fibromyalgia, combating fatigue is an ongoing battle. No matter how many times a week you exercise or how healthy a diet you follow, if you are overextended, you will wear yourself out. You can lessen your fatigue by setting priorities and conserving your strength for the things you value most.

Use the priority sheet on the next page to help you understand what is important to you and how you can make adjustments in your life to enjoy the things you like to do. A sample priority sheet is shown below.

Priority Sheet Sample

Photocopy this worksheet and make a list of basic priority questions, and fill in your own responses to determine what activities are most vital to you.

WHAT IS MOST IMPORTANT TO YOU?

My family

Feeling normal

WHAT ACTIVITIES ARE RELEVANT TO THE PRIORITIES YOU'VE IDENTIFIED?

Going on "dates" with my husband

Going to movies with kids

Yoga!

WHAT MUST YOU ACCOMPLISH?

Housework

Going to kids' games

WHAT CAN YOU ASK OTHER PEOPLE TO DO?

Ask kids to help more with chores

Ask my husband to make or bring home dinner once a week

WHAT CAN BE MODIFIED OR SIMPLIFIED?

Simpler meals — leftovers

Break chores out across entire week — not just one day

ACTIVITY

Priority Sheet

Photocopy this worksheet and make a list of basic priority questions, and fill in your own responses to determine what activities are most vital to you.

WHAT IS MOST IMPORTANT TO YOU?

_____
_____
_____
_____

WHAT ACTIVITIES ARE RELEVANT TO THE PRIORITIES YOU'VE IDENTIFIED?

_____
_____
_____
_____
_____

WHAT MUST YOU ACCOMPLISH?

_____
_____
_____
_____

WHAT CAN YOU ELIMINATE?

_____
_____
_____
_____

WHAT CAN YOU ASK OTHER PEOPLE TO DO?

_____
_____
_____
_____
_____
_____

WHAT CAN BE MODIFIED OR SIMPLIFIED?

_____
_____
_____
_____
_____
_____

WHAT CAN YOU SAY NO TO?

_____
_____
_____
_____
_____

Pace Yourself

No matter how well you prioritize your activities, if you try to do too much at once, you are going to wear yourself out. That is why you must pace yourself and recognize your limits. Answer these questions to see if you are doing what you can.

❑ YES ❑ NO Are you taking breaks between or during tasks before you get tired? A ratio of 10 minutes of rest for every 50 minutes of activity works well for many people.

❑ YES ❑ NO Do you alternate light and heavy tasks? Do the toughest jobs when you are feeling best. Divide big jobs into little ones.

❑ YES ❑ NO Are you taking it slowly? Don't rush. You are a more efficient worker if you do your activity at a comfortable pace.

❑ YES ❑ NO Do you avoid activities that will tap all of your energy? Learn to say no to activities that will drain you of energy and cause fatigue.

Problem-Solving for Fatigue

Does your fatigue get in the way of doing things you've always done? Whether it's a chore, like cleaning the house, or something you enjoy, like gardening, finding simple solutions may help you get back to doing the everyday things you miss.

Photocopy and use the worksheet on the following page to write down your causes for fatigue and then write down possible solutions that may help you avoid becoming fatigued. A sample is shown below.

Fatigue Problem-Solving Sample

CAUSE OF FATIGUE	POSSIBLE SOLUTIONS
Getting up early for work	Ask about flex-time Go to bed earlier Shower at night

ACTIVITY

Fatigue Problem-Solving

CAUSE OF FATIGUE	POSSIBLE SOLUTIONS

Problem-Solving for Fatigue

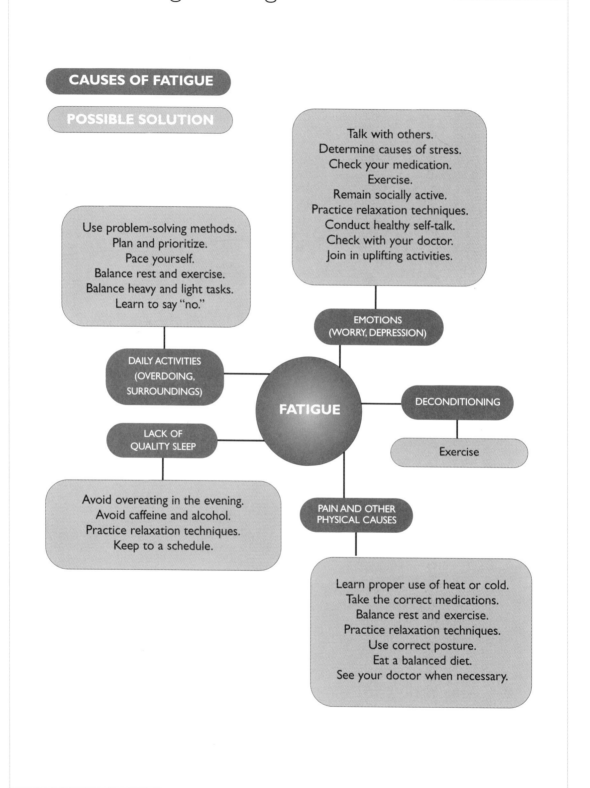

CAUSES OF FATIGUE

POSSIBLE SOLUTION

Talk with others.
Determine causes of stress.
Check your medication.
Exercise.
Remain socially active.
Practice relaxation techniques.
Conduct healthy self-talk.
Check with your doctor.
Join in uplifting activities.

Use problem-solving methods.
Plan and prioritize.
Pace yourself.
Balance rest and exercise.
Balance heavy and light tasks.
Learn to say "no."

EMOTIONS
(WORRY, DEPRESSION)

DAILY ACTIVITIES
(OVERDOING,
SURROUNDINGS)

FATIGUE

DECONDITIONING

LACK OF
QUALITY SLEEP

Exercise

Avoid overeating in the evening.
Avoid caffeine and alcohol.
Practice relaxation techniques.
Keep to a schedule.

PAIN AND OTHER
PHYSICAL CAUSES

Learn proper use of heat or cold.
Take the correct medications.
Balance rest and exercise.
Practice relaxation techniques.
Use correct posture.
Eat a balanced diet.
See your doctor when necessary.

GOOD LIVING
GOOD LIVING
GOOD LIVING
GOOD LIVING
GOOD LIVING
GOOD LIVING
GOOD LIVING
GOOD LIVING
GOOD LIVING
GOOD LIVING

CHAPTER 12:

Resting Well

Getting a good night's rest is a challenge for people with fibromyalgia. Abnormal sleep patterns are present in most people with fibromyalgia. The side effects of poor sleep worsen the other symptoms of fibromyalgia – from pain and fatigue to cognitive dysfunction.

The activities in this chapter will help you identify sleeping problems and develop better sleeping habits.

How Well Do You Sleep?

Sleep disturbance is one of the most common and troubling symptoms of fibromyalgia. Without restful sleep, people with fibromyalgia are more prone to fatigue, pain and concentration problems.

What is your biggest problem with sleep? Check the boxes below.

❑ I can't fall asleep at bedtime. It takes hours for me to fall asleep.

❑ I rarely sleep throughout the night. I wake up on and off throughout the night.

❑ I wake up in the middle of the night and can't fall back to sleep.

❑ I sleep throughout the night but still feel tired when I wake up in the morning.

Sleep Diary Sample

Fill out days 1-7 below	I went to bed last night at:	I got out of bed this morning at:	Last night I fell asleep in:	I woke up during the night: (Number of times)	When I woke up for the day, I felt: (Check one)	Last night I slept for a total of: (Number of times)	My sleep was disturbed by:
COMPLETE IN MORNING							
DAY 1 day **Mon.** date **4/8**	11:15 (p.m.)/a.m.	7:30 p.m./(a.m.)	30 Minutes	1 Times	_ Refreshed ✓ Somewhat Refreshed _ Fatigued	6½ Hours	bathroom
DAY 2 day **Tues.** date **4/9**	11 (p.m.)/a.m.	7:45 p.m./(a.m.)	60 Minutes	2 Times	_ Refreshed _ Somewhat Refreshed ✓ Fatigued	5 Hours	don't know— jumpy feeling
DAY 3 day **Wed.** date **4/10**	11:45 (p.m.)/a.m.	7:30 p.m./(a.m.)	30 Minutes	0 Times	_ Refreshed ✓ Somewhat Refreshed _ Fatigued	7½ Hours	nothing— took Ambien
DAY 4 day **Thurs.** date **4/11**	11:30 (p.m.)/a.m.	5:30 p.m./(a.m.)	60 Minutes	1 Times	_ Refreshed _ Somewhat Refreshed ✓ Fatigued	5 Hours	worried about busy day

ACTIVITY

Keep a Sleep Diary

Photocopy this worksheet and use it to record your sleep patterns at night and share it with your doctor. Together you can work together to develop a treatment plan that works for you.

Fill out days 1-7 below	I went to bed last night at:	I got out of bed this morning at:	Last night I fell asleep in:	I woke up during the night: (Number of times)	When I woke up for the day, I felt: (Check one)	Last night I slept for a total of: (Number of times)	My sleep was disturbed by:
	COMPLETE IN MORNING						
DAY 1 day _____ date _____	p.m./a.m.	p.m./a.m.	Minutes	Times	_ Refreshed _ Somewhat Refreshed _ Fatigued	Hours	_____ _____
DAY 2 day _____ date _____	p.m./a.m.	p.m./a.m.	Minutes	Times	_ Refreshed _ Somewhat Refreshed _ Fatigued	Hours	_____ _____
DAY 3 day _____ date _____	p.m./a.m.	p.m./a.m.	Minutes	Times	_ Refreshed _ Somewhat Refreshed _ Fatigued	Hours	_____ _____
DAY 4 day _____ date _____	p.m./a.m.	p.m./a.m.	Minutes	Times	_ Refreshed _ Somewhat Refreshed _ Fatigued	Hours	_____ _____
DAY 5 day _____ date _____	p.m./a.m.	p.m./a.m.	Minutes	Times	_ Refreshed _ Somewhat Refreshed _ Fatigued	Hours	_____ _____
DAY 6 day _____ date _____	p.m./a.m.	p.m./a.m.	Minutes	Times	_ Refreshed _ Somewhat Refreshed _ Fatigued	Hours	_____ _____
DAY 7 day _____ date _____	p.m./a.m.	p.m./a.m.	Minutes	Times	_ Refreshed _ Somewhat Refreshed _ Fatigued	Hours	_____ _____

continued on page 140

Fill out days 1-7 below	COMPLETE AT END OF DAY				
	I consumed caffeinated drinks in the: (e.g. coffee, tea, soda)	I exercised at least 20 minutes in the:	Approximately 2-3 hours before going to bed, I consumed:	Medications I took during the day: (List name of medication/drug)	About 1 hour before going to sleep, I did the following activity: (List activity: e.g. watch TV, work, read)
DAY 1 day _____ date _____	__ Morning __ Afternoon __ About 2-3 hours before going to bed __ Not applicable	__ Morning __ Afternoon __ About 2-3 hours before going to bed __ Not applicable	__ Alcohol __ A heavy meal __ Not applicable	_____ _____ _____	_____ _____ _____
DAY 2 day _____ date _____	__ Morning __ Afternoon __ About 2-3 hours before going to bed __ Not applicable	__ Morning __ Afternoon __ About 2-3 hours before going to bed __ Not applicable	__ Alcohol __ A heavy meal __ Not applicable	_____ _____ _____	_____ _____ _____
DAY 3 day _____ date _____	__ Morning __ Afternoon __ About 2-3 hours before going to bed __ Not applicable	__ Morning __ Afternoon __ About 2-3 hours before going to bed __ Not applicable	__ Alcohol __ A heavy meal __ Not applicable	_____ _____ _____	_____ _____ _____
DAY 4 day _____ date _____	__ Morning __ Afternoon __ About 2-3 hours before going to bed __ Not applicable	__ Morning __ Afternoon __ About 2-3 hours before going to bed __ Not applicable	__ Alcohol __ A heavy meal __ Not applicable	_____ _____ _____	_____ _____ _____
DAY 5 day _____ date _____	__ Morning __ Afternoon __ About 2-3 hours before going to bed __ Not applicable	__ Morning __ Afternoon __ About 2-3 hours before going to bed __ Not applicable	__ Alcohol __ A heavy meal __ Not applicable	_____ _____ _____	_____ _____ _____
DAY 6 day _____ date _____	__ Morning __ Afternoon __ About 2-3 hours before going to bed __ Not applicable	__ Morning __ Afternoon __ About 2-3 hours before going to bed __ Not applicable	__ Alcohol __ A heavy meal __ Not applicable	_____ _____ _____	_____ _____ _____
DAY 7 day _____ date _____	__ Morning __ Afternoon __ About 2-3 hours before going to bed __ Not applicable	__ Morning __ Afternoon __ About 2-3 hours before going to bed __ Not applicable	__ Alcohol __ A heavy meal __ Not applicable	_____ _____ _____	_____ _____ _____

* Reprinted with permission from the National Sleep Foundation; www.nsf.org.

Eliminate the Factors That Disturb Sleep

Researchers continue to investigate the correlation between fibromyalgia and sleep disturbance. In the meantime, doctors will prescribe doses of exercise, relaxation and medication to help you get the necessary rest you need to stave off the pain and fatigue associated with your condition.

However, there may be some factors in your life that contribute to your sleep problems that are not associated with fibromyalgia. Could the following factors be interfering with your sleep? Check the boxes below.

❏ YES ❏ NO Do you take medications that could interfere with sleep? Talk to your doctor about all medications you take, even over-the-counter medications, such as cold medicines. Your doctor may be able to help you adjust the times you take medications to best help you get the sleep you need.

❏ YES ❏ NO Are you consuming too much caffeine? Avoid caffeine at night. Consider drinking decaffeinated coffee, tea, or soda. People, especially older people, develop a progressive sensitivity to caffeine.

❏ YES ❏ NO Do you eat foods that disrupt sleep? Avoid eating too much or eating foods that can cause stomach distress at bedtime. Spicy or greasy foods can cause indigestion that can prevent you from sleeping soundly.

❏ YES ❏ NO Do you take in a lot of fluids before bedtime? Drinking too much fluid before bedtime may cause you to have to get up in the middle of the night to go to the bathroom. You may have difficulty returning to sleep.

❏ YES ❏ NO Do you smoke? There are myriad reasons for you to quit smoking. One of them is to help you sleep. Smoking to relax is a common misconception. In fact, nicotine stimulates the nervous system, making falling asleep more difficult.

❏ YES ❏ NO Do you drink alcohol? People often believe that alcohol, which is a depressant, will help them sleep. However, although alcohol consumption may help you doze off, once the effects have worn off and your body has processed the alcohol, you may wake up and have difficulty returning to sleep.

❏ YES ❏ NO Are you stressed out? Stress – both good and bad – can interfere with your ability to fall asleep. Learn some relaxation exercises to help you release anxiety and get the rest you need.

❏ YES ❏ NO Do you have physical problems that interfere with sleep? Talk to your doctor if you are often in pain or have a physical condition that disrupts sleep, such as restless legs syndrome.

Medications That Promote Sleep

Not all experts agree on the need for medication to help people sleep or the type of medication that works best. Nor is the best medication for one person necessarily the best for all. In general, however, here are some drugs experts recommend or prescribe to help their patients ease their pain and get some sleep.

Drug Category	Examples	How They May Help	Things To Consider
Analgesics	acetaminophen (*Tylenol*), propoxyphene (*Darvon*)	Ease the pain of fibro-myalgia, which can make it difficult to fall or stay asleep	While acetaminophen is safe if taken as directed, narcotic analgesics can be habit-forming. Many doctors will not prescribe them for long-term pain.
Nonsteroidal Anti-Inflammatory Drugs (NSAIDs)	ibuprofen (*Advil, Motrin*), naproxen (*Naprosyn, Naprelan*), ketoprofen (*Orudis, Oruvail*)	Ease the pain of fibromyal-gia, which can make it diffi-cult to fall or stay asleep	Some pain-relief preparations contain antihistamines that can make you drowsy; others contain caffeine or other ingredients that can make sleep-ing more difficult. Ask your doctor which NSAID is right for you. When purchasing over-the-counter NSAIDs, look for hidden ingredients.
Tricyclic Antidepressants	amitriptyline (*Elavil*), cyclobenzaprine (*Flexeril*), doxepin (*Adapin, Sinequan*), Nortriptyline (*Aventyl, Pamelor*)	Ease pain, relax muscles and increase deep sleep	Tricyclic antidepressants are among the most widely studied and pre-scribed medications for fibromyalgia-related sleep problems.
Pyrazolopyrimidines	zalepan (*Sonata*)	Offer short-term assis-tance for people who have trouble falling asleep or returning to sleep	This fast-acting drug takes only 20 minutes for most people to fall asleep. Because the effects last only an hour, pyrazolopyrimidines are pre-scribed for people who cannot take long-acting sleep aids.
Benzodiazepines	tamezepam (*Restoril*), lorezepam (*Ativan*), clonazepam (*Klonopin*)	Increase slow wave sleep and control periodic limb movement and restless legs syndrome, which can interfere with sleep	Benzodiazepines may cause depres-sion and addiction, so your doctor may prescribe them along with an antidepressant. Because of side effects, some doctors will not prescribe them long-term or they may prescribe them for use on alternate nights.
Central Nervous System Depressants	zolpidem (*Ambien*), trazodone (*Desyrel*)	Enable most people to get a full eight hours of sleep	Many doctors will not prescribe zolpi-dem for chronic sleeplessness. Long-term use may cause the medication to lose its effectiveness.

Please note that this is not a comprehensive list of medications for sleep and fibromyalgia. Your doctor may prescribe others. There are many drugs in each of these categories; the drugs listed here are only a sample. Some drugs in each category provide more benefits for certain problems than do others. The inclusion of a particular drug here does not imply that it works better than others in its class. The Arthritis Foundation does not endorse any medication or particular brand of medication.

Seven Tips for Better Sleep

Getting a good night's sleep isn't all a matter of getting the right medication. If you're not sleeping well, there are plenty of things you can do on your own to help get your share of shut-eye. Here are seven suggestions from the experts:

1. EXERCISE REGULARLY.

Exercise increases blood flow through the muscles and increases slow-wave sleep. But avoid exercising too close to bedtime. For some people, that has a stimulating effect.

2. TAKE A WARM BATH.

Like exercise, warm water can increase circulation. It can also relax sore muscles, making sleep more likely.

3. LEARN TO RELAX.

Relaxation techniques, such as breathing or muscle tension-and-release exercises, can help ease pain and take your mind off worries that may be keeping you awake at night.

4. KEEP IT COOL.

A cool, dark room is conducive to sleep.

5. SKIP THE NAP.

While it may be tempting to make up for missed sleep in the afternoon, doing so can make it difficult to get to sleep at night, perpetuating the vicious cycle.

6. CUT OUT THE CAFFEINE.

Particularly if consumed in the afternoon or evening, caffeine can interfere with nighttime sleep. So can nicotine and alcohol.

7. CHECK YOUR MEDICATIONS.

Certain medications can keep you awake at night. If you think a medication might be interfering with your sleep, don't stop taking it without first consulting your doctor. It may be possible to change the dose or the timing of medication to minimize its effects on your much-needed rest.

Restless Legs Syndrome: Ants in Your Pants?

As if they didn't have enough problems sleeping, many people with fibromyalgia also have a condition known as restless legs syndrome (RLS). How do you distinguish RLS from other sleep-preventing symptoms? Ask yourself the following questions:

❑ YES ❑ NO

Do you experience bothersome sensations in your legs that give you the irresistible urge to move?

❑ YES ❑ NO

Are the symptoms at their worst when you are at rest and lessened with voluntary movement?

❑ YES ❑ NO

Are the symptoms at their worst at night, especially when lying down?

❑ YES ❑ NO

Do your toes, feet or legs move involuntarily when you are sitting or lying down in the evening?

If you think you have RLS, talk to your doctor. In addition to instructing you to follow the standard sleep suggestions offered on page 143, your doctor may be able to prescribe a medication to help calm your twitchy limbs.

GOOD LIVING
GOOD LIVING
GOOD LIVING
GOOD LIVING
GOOD LIVING
GOOD LIVING
GOOD LIVING
GOOD LIVING
GOOD LIVING

CHAPTER 13:

Achieving Relaxation

The stresses of everyday living are difficult for anyone. For people living with fibromyalgia, those stresses are compounded. Unless you have healthy outlets for relieving stress, your fibromyalgia symptoms can get worse. How you achieve relaxation depends on the stresses you face day-to-day and how your body reacts to stress. Use the activities in this chapter to help you identify the stresses in your life and find a healthy means for achieving relaxation.

Stress Signals: Listen to Your Body

Your body has ways of alerting you that you are becoming overstressed. Look for the signals your body gives you that you are feeling stressed.

- Headaches. Do you feel tension in shoulders, neck or arm muscles? Do your shoulders hunch? Are you clenching your teeth?

- Stomach upset. Is your stomach knotted? Do you feel like you have butterflies? Are you experiencing loss of appetite? Do you have diarrhea or constipation?

- Emotional reactions. Are you feeling anxious, moody, angry or hopeless? Do you have low self-esteem? Are you having problems concentrating? Do you feel depressed?

- Sleeping problems. Do you have trouble falling asleep or do you wake up too early? Do you wake up in the middle of the night and then have trouble falling back to sleep? Are you sleeping too much? Do you experience troubling dreams?

- Other signs. Do you have chronic fatigue? Do you have cold, clammy hands? Is your heart pounding or does your chest feel tight or heavy? Do you have dry mouth?

How Does Your Body React to Stress?

Understanding how your body reacts to stress physically and emotionally will help you learn how to manage your stress and break the destructive cycle. How does your body react to stress? Do you have:

❑ YES ❑ NO Headaches

❑ YES ❑ NO Stomach distress, ulcers

❑ YES ❑ NO High blood pressure

❑ YES ❑ NO Muscle tension, back pain and other types of pain

❑ YES ❑ NO Chronic fatigue

❑ YES ❑ NO Restlessness, irritability, frustration

❑ YES ❑ NO Decreased zest for life, worry, fear, depression

❑ YES ❑ NO Difficulty making decisions, forgetfulness

❑ YES ❑ NO Increased use of alcohol, cigarettes or drugs

❑ YES ❑ NO Eating and sleeping problems

❑ YES ❑ NO Disease flares

Stress Busters

Here are eight simple ways you can relieve stress:

- Relax in a warm bath.
- Sit quietly and concentrate on deep breathing for 5 to 10 minutes.
- Drink a soothing cup of herbal tea.
- Read a good book.
- Work a crossword or other type of puzzle.
- Write your thoughts and feelings in a journal.
- Exercise – take a walk or do some stretching.
- Listen to your favorite soothing music.
- Do something creative, like painting, drawing, sewing or cooking.

Recognize Your Stress Signals

Identifying what causes your stress will help you and your health-care team discover ways to manage your stress. Keep a record of your stresses and share them with your health-care providers. Photocopy and use the stress diary on the following page. A sample stress diary is shown below.

Sample Stress Diary

DATE	CAUSE OF STRESS	TIME	PHYSICAL SYMPTOMS	EMOTIONAL SYMPTOMS
10/26	presentation at work	10 a.m.	stomach upset fatigue	worry fear
10/27	traffic	5 p.m.	headache	anger
10/29	dinner with client	8 p.m.	stomach upset	nervous

ACTIVITY

Keeping a Stress Diary

Record the events in your life that cause stress, as well as any physical or emotional symptoms that result. After one week, look for patterns in symptoms, determine what causes them and make life adjustments.

DATE	CAUSE OF STRESS	TIME	PHYSICAL SYMPTOMS	EMOTIONAL SYMPTOMS

Change What You Can

Once you've recognized the causes of stress in your life, you can take steps to change those stressors. Use these strategies to reduce the stresses that agitate your fibromyalgia.

- **Set goals.** Do you keep track of the things you want to accomplish on a daily basis?

- **List your priorities.** What needs to be done immediately? What can be done later? What can be eliminated?

- **Eliminate daily hassles.** Can you scale back your work hours? Can you avoid people who annoy or stress you? Can you delegate some of your daily workload to other family members?

- **Let uplifting activities outnumber hassles.** Can you incorporate more of the activity from the Uplifts Scale (page 152) and eliminate some from the Hassles Scale (page 153)?

- **Pamper yourself.** Do you take time do the things you enjoy? Do you save time to just take care of you?

- **Plan for special events.** Do you give yourself plenty of time to prepare for the holidays? Do you shop for gifts when you feel well? Do you plan ahead and accept help when you are entertaining?

- **Acknowledge major life events as stress.** Do you realize that exciting events like a wedding, graduation, getting a new job or even taking a vacation can be stressful? Can you better prepare for them?

- **Learn to say no.** Have you lost the guilty feeling of telling people no when you are asked to volunteer?

- **Think "win/win."** Do you come up with compromising solutions to the problems and conflicts you have in your daily life?

- **Learn to accept the things you can't change.** Are you being realistic about your limitations? Do you understand that you can't change other people or all situations? Can you be flexible when necessary?

ACTIVITY

Uplifts Scale

Uplifts are events that make you feel good. They are sources of your contentment, satisfaction and joy. Photocopy this chart and put a check by any events that may have made you feel good in the last <u>month</u>. **Optional:** Rate how <u>strongly</u> you feel that each of the following uplifts improves your spirits on a scale of 1 to 3 (1 = somewhat strongly; 2 = moderately strongly and 3 = extremely strongly). Then add up your total score. Compare to the score on your Hassles Scale on the next page. Aim for getting an Uplifts score that is at least twice your total Hassles score

1. Getting enough sleep	23. Spending time with friends
2. Being lucky	24. Buying things for yourself or home
3. Saving money	25. Home pleasing you
4. Not working	26. Giving or getting a present
5. Having a pleasant conversation	27. Traveling
6. Feeling healthy	28. Doing yardwork
7. Being pregnant	29. Making a friend
8. Visiting, phoning or writing someone	30. Getting unexpected money
9. Relating well with your spouse or lover	31. Dreaming
10. Completing a task	32. Pets
11. Being efficient; meeting responsibilities	33. Children's accomplishments
12. Cutting down on smoking	34. Things going well at work
13. Cutting down on drinking	35. Making decisions
14. Losing weight	36. Confronting someone
15. Good sex	37. Being alone
16. Friendly neighbors	38. Knowing your job is secure
17. Eating out	39. Feeling safe in your neighborhood
18. Using drugs or alcohol	40. Fixing something
19. Having plenty of energy	41. Meeting a challenge
20. Relaxing	42. Flirting
21. Having the "right" amount of things to do	Other uplifts, not mentioned yet:
22. Being creative	43.

ACTIVITY

Hassles Scale

Hassles are irritations that can range from minor annoyances to fairly major pressures. Listed here are a number of ways in which a person can feel hassled. Photocopy this chart, then go through the list and put a check by those hassles that have happened to you in the past month. Optional: Rate how severe each hassle has been on a scale of 1-3 (1 = somewhat severe; 2 = moderately severe; and 3 = extremely severe). Then, add up your total score. Compare the score on your Uplifts Scale (see previous page). Aim for getting an Uplifts score that is at least twice your total Hassles score.

1. Misplacing things	23. Not getting enough sleep
2. Trouble with neighbors	24. Problems with your children
3. Social obligations	25. Problems with your parents
4. Health of family member	26. Problems with your spouse or lover
5. Concerns about debts	27. Too much to do
6. Smoking too much	28. Work unchallenging
7. Drinking too much	29. Legal problems
8. Trouble relaxing	30. Concerns about weight
9. Trouble making decisions	31. Not enough energy
10. Problems with people at work	32. Feeling conflict over what to do
11. Customers/clients giving you a hard time	33. Not enough time for family
12. Home maintenance	34. Property, investments, taxes
13. Concerns about job security	35. Yardwork
14. Don't like current job	36. Concerns about news
15. Bored	37. Crime
16. Lonely	38. Traffic
17. Fear of confrontation	39. Pollution
18. Illness	Other hassles not mentioned yet:
19. Physical appearance	40.
20. Problems at work	41.
21. Car trouble	42.
22. Rising prices	43.

GOOD LIVING
GOOD LIVING
GOOD LIVING
GOOD LIVING
GOOD LIVING
GOOD LIVING
GOOD LIVING
GOOD LIVING
GOOD LIVING

CHAPTER 14:

Losses and Gains

I t's OK to mourn the loss of the person you were before you were diagnosed with fibromyalgia. And it's OK to mourn the loss of those things you may no longer be able to do. But it's not OK to wallow in your grief. Grieving is natural, but you must also learn to deal with your grief and move on to the business of living.

How Do You Deal With Your Grief?

Grief is a natural response to loss. And for people with fibromyalgia, those losses vary. For some they may be physical, while for others they may social or personal. How you grieve also varies.

Dealing with your grief – whether you try to work through it or just accept it – will help you feel better about yourself and your fibromyalgia. Use the checklist below to see which methods you use to deal with your feelings of grief.

❑ YES ❑ NO

Do you permit yourself to experience your feelings? Give yourself permission to be sad or angry. Don't deny yourself these normal emotions of the grieving process. But don't let them take over your life.

❑ YES ❑ NO

Do you know what triggers your fears and emotions? Do a little self-discovery to find out what emotional support you need that you aren't getting and what causes you to feel the way you do. Limit the time you spend with people who make you feel uncomfortable.

❑ YES ❑ NO

Are you able to express your fears and feelings and then let them go? Don't keep your feelings bottled up. Let them out. Talk to a friend, write in a journal, scream in the shower. But don't dwell in those feelings. Learn to let them go.

❑ YES ❑ NO

Can you find meaning in your experiences with fibromyalgia? Think about the positive things that have occurred as a result of your fibromyalgia. For example, have you developed new hobbies, made new friends, reassessed your priorities or strengthened your relationship with God or spirituality? The Losses and Discovery List on page 158 can help.

Possible Grief Responses

SHOCK AND DENIAL: "NO! IT CAN'T BE TRUE!" Denial is a protective buffer, allowing you to replace anxious thoughts with more hopeful ones. Denial buys time for you to mobilize other coping techniques and face your losses at a manageable pace. This stage is usually temporary, but if you can't accept your diagnosis, you won't be able to fight your condition.

BARGAINING: "LET'S MAKE A DEAL." You may find yourself making secret promises — for example, "I'll become a better person" if fate or a higher power sends a cure. Or you may begin an endless cycle of seeking other medical opinions and trying unproven remedies. This process is yet another "time-buying" stage before acceptance.

ANGER: "WHY ME?" Anger, rage, envy and resentment are all common responses to bad news like a diagnosis of fibromyalgia. You may express your anger by criticizing your doctor, family or friends. You may put off necessary chores or treatments, or sink into depression. You may feel cheated by fate or a higher power. But if you don't move beyond this stage, you can become extremely irritable and quarrelsome.

GUILT: "I DESERVED IT." Next, you may blame yourself for having fibromyalgia. ("I should have been a better person; I should have taken better care of myself," and so on.) You may begin to think of yourself as a burden to others. And just as you view your illness as a personal failure, you think if you try harder to do more, you'll feel better.

SADNESS AND DEPRESSION: "I WILL MISS BEING ABLE TO . . . ." This stage is a natural part of saying goodbye to lost roles and abilities. It usually gets better in time. However, if this stage persists, depression will set in as a lingering sense of despair and worthlessness. It can also be a quiet cover for anger, anxiety or guilt. Depression persists until negative thinking is changed.

FEAR AND UNCERTAINTY: "WHAT ELSE WILL HAPPEN?" Also natural responses to fibromyalgia's unpredictable variations, fear and uncertainty themselves may cause muscle tension, increased heart rate, stomach distress and trembling. Signs that you're stuck in this stage include anticipating the future with fear and anxiety, worrying about the next bad bout even during periods of good health, or feeling helpless or out of control over your health from day to day.

LONELINESS AND ISOLATION: "NO ONE UNDERSTANDS." Curtailing your activities can lead to fewer social contacts. Also, some friends may withdraw because they don't know how to help. Family members may become emotionally exhausted. All these factors can lead to isolation and loneliness if you don't work at broadening your support system and maintaining contact with the outside world.

RECONCILIATION AND ACCEPTANCE: "I MAY HAVE FIBROMYALGIA BUT. . . ." Acceptance is the final stage of grief, but the first sign you're ready to build a new life. Once you are able to let go of the past and the person you were before you developed fibromyalgia, you can get on with your recovery.

ACTIVITY

Losses and Discovery List

Photocopy this worksheet and use the blanks below to list the losses you've experienced as a result of fibromyalgia. In the space provided, list the positive things that you may have discovered as a result.

Examples:

Loss: I have lost my independence.

Discovery: I have learned to be comfortable letting other people help.

Loss: I no longer sleep through the night.

Discovery: I feel healthier when I don't drink or eat anything with caffeine. I hardly miss it.

Loss: _____

_____

Discovery: _____

_____

Loss: _____

_____

Discovery: _____

_____

Loss: _____

_____

Discovery: _____

_____

Use Self-Talk

The conversations you have with yourself in your head constitute self-talk. There are two kinds of self-talk: healthy and unhealthy. Healthy self-talk serves as your personal cheering section ("I look great today"). Unhealthy self-talk comes from responding to situations with automatic negative thoughts ("Why do I always say dumb things?").

In order to turn your negative thoughts into healthy self-talk, you need to pay attention to your thoughts throughout the day. Use the Thoughts Diary on the following page to record your negative thoughts and come up with suggestions to change them into positive, healthy self-talk.

Getting Self-Talk To Work for You

- Write down self-defeating thoughts.

- Do a "reality check." Ask:
  - Are there other ways of looking at this situation?
  - What am I afraid will occur?
  - How do I know that this outcome will indeed happen?
  - What evidence do I have that this outcome will happen?
  - Is there evidence that contradicts this conclusion?
  - What coping resources are available?
  - Have I only had failures in the past, or were there times I did okay?
  - There are times when I don't do as well as I would like, but other times I do, so what are the differences between those times?

- Change self-defeating thoughts to helpful self-talk.

- Mentally rehearse healthy self-talk.

- Practice healthy self-talk in real situations.

- Be patient – it takes time for new patterns of thinking to become automatic.

Thoughts Diary

To appreciate the power of your self-talk and the part it plays in your emotional life, make your own thoughts diary. Photocopy this diary and make a notation each time you experience an unpleasant emotion. Include everything you tell yourself to keep the emotion going.

Date	Unpleasant Emotion	Situation	Self-Talk	Rational Response

Are You Depressed?

Every now and then, we all experience a few depressive symptoms. Sometimes the pressures of work, home, family and fibromyalgia become too much to bear. But those feelings fade, and you pick yourself up and go back to the business of living.

However, for some people, shaking those depressive symptoms is not so easy. If you think you may be depressed, take the self-test on the next page to find out.

Are You at Risk?

Some people are at higher risk for depression at certain times in their lives or under certain conditions. Use the checklist below to see if you are at risk.

❏ YES ❏ NO Have you had a previous episode of depression?

❏ YES ❏ NO Did your previous depressive episode occur before age 40?

❏ YES ❏ NO Do you have a medical condition?

❏ YES ❏ NO Have you recently given birth?

❏ YES ❏ NO Are you without a support network?

❏ YES ❏ NO Have you recently experienced a stressful life event (positive or negative)?

❏ YES ❏ NO Do you abuse alcohol or drugs?

❏ YES ❏ NO Do you have a family history of depression-related disorders?

❏ YES ❏ NO Have you experienced only partial relief from a previous episode of depression?

Depression: A Self-Test

Experiencing one or more of these depressive symptoms every now and then is a normal part of life. If a certain number of these symptoms have been bothering you for weeks or years, you may have a depressive disorder and should consult your doctor with this list in hand. See the results below.

GROUP 1:

Are you experiencing at least one of the following nearly every day?

❑ apathy, or loss of interest in things you used to enjoy, including sex

❑ sadness, blues or irritability

GROUP 2:

In addition, are you experiencing any of the following?

❑ feeling slowed down or restless

❑ feeling worthless or guilty

❑ changes in appetite or a substantial weight loss or gain

❑ problems concentrating, thinking, remembering or making decisions

❑ trouble falling asleep or sleeping too much

❑ loss of energy, feeling tired all the time

GROUP 3:

And what about the following symptoms? These symptoms are not used to diagnose depressive disorders, but often occur with them.

❑ headaches*

❑ other aches and pains*

❑ digestive problems*

❑ sexual problems*

❑ feeling pessimistic or hopeless

❑ being anxious or worried

❑ low self-esteem

RESULTS:

If you have several symptoms, talk to your physician. (Note: Your physician may refer you to a mental health professional if you need more help.) You may be clinically depressed if you experience at least one of the symptoms in Group 1 and at least four of the symptoms in Group 2 nearly every day for at least two weeks.

You may have chronic depression if you experience at least one of the symptoms in Group 1 and at least two of the symptoms in Group 2 nearly every day for at least two years.

*These are potential indications of depression only if not caused by another disease or by medication.

Choosing a Counselor

Whether you are depressed or just feel frustrated, a professional counselor can help you come to grips with your feelings and work on ways to improve your feelings. Don't let the frustration of finding a helpful counselor prevent you from getting the help you need. The following tips will help you find someone suitable for you.

- Look for credentials. Do they have appropriate mental-health education and training? Are they affiliated with any professional organizations? Do they have a license or other certification?

- Look for experience. Do they have experience working with people with fibromyalgia or other chronic diseases?

- Look for referrals. Do you know anyone they have helped? Do you know of other health professionals who recommend them?

- Look for a good fit. Do you feel comfortable with them? Do they make you feel at ease?

Where To Find Help

The following organizations offer general information on depressive disorders, mental illness and finding a therapist. Some organizations also have a referral service to help you find a credentialed therapist in your area.

American Association for Marriage and Family Therapy, 703/838-9808; www.aamft.org.

American Psychiatric Association, 703/907-73000; www.psych.org.

American Psychological Association, 800/374-2721; www.apa.org.

National Alliance for the Mentally Ill, 800/950-6264; www.nami.org.

National Association of Social Workers, 800/742-4089; www.naswdc.org.

National Depressive and Manic-Depressive Association, 800/826-3632; www.dbsalliance.org.

National Mental Health Association, 800/969-6642; www.nmha.org.

GOOD LIVING
GOOD LIVING
GOOD LIVING
GOOD LIVING
GOOD LIVING
GOOD LIVING
GOOD LIVING
GOOD LIVING
GOOD LIVING

CHAPTER 15:

Money Matters

With or without fibromyalgia, getting a financial check-up is as important as getting a health check-up. When you have fibromyalgia, however, it is especially important to examine your finances. You must see how financially prepared you are to handle health-related expenses. The activities in this chapter will help you conduct a financial inventory and set financial goals for yourself.

Take a Financial Inventory

Before you can make financial goals for yourself, you need to assess your current financial situation. You can do this by evaluating your net worth, which is subtracting the amount of your liabilities (what you owe) from the value of your assets (what you own). Use the following worksheets to determine your net worth.

ACTIVITY

Your Assets, Liabilities and Net Worth

Photocopy this worksheet and use it to take an inventory of your (and your partner's) assets and liabilities.

ASSETS	NAME/ACCOUNT #	VALUE
Home		
Spouse/partner		
Mine		
Ours		
Vehicle(s)		
Spouse/partner		
Mine		
Ours		
Checking Accounts		
Spouse/partner		
Mine		
Ours		
Savings Accounts		
Spouse/partner		
Mine		
Ours		
Investments		
Spouse/partner		
Mine		
Ours		

ASSETS	NAME/ACCOUNT #	VALUE
Retirement Plan(s) [IRAs, 401(k)s, 403(b)s]		
Spouse/partner		
Mine		
Ours		
Furniture		
Spouse/partner		
Mine		
Ours		
Artwork/Collectibles		
Spouse/partner		
Mine		
Ours		
Jewelry		
Spouse/partner		
Mine		
Ours		
Rental Property or Time-Shares		
Spouse/partner		
Mine		
Ours		
Business		
Spouse/partner		
Mine		
Ours		
Other		
Spouse/partner		
Mine		
Ours		

Your Assets, Liabilities and Net Worth

LIABILITIES (DEBTS)	NAME/ACCOUNT #	AMOUNT OWED
Home Mortgage		
Spouse/partner		
Mine		
Ours		
Car Payment(s)		
Spouse/partner		
Mine		
Ours		
Credit Card Debt		
Spouse/partner		
Mine		
Ours		
Other Loans		
Spouse/partner		
Mine		
Ours		
Totals:		
Spouse/partner		
My Assets		
Our Assets		
Spouse/partner Liabilities		
My Liabilities		
Our Liabilities		

Spouse's/Partner's Net Worth (assets minus liabilities) $ _____

My Net Worth $ _____

Our Net Worth $ _____

Create a Spending Plan

Spending plan is a nice word for a budget. Everyone hates budgets, but if you want to find ways to save your money and cut expenses, you'll need to develop one. It will help you to know how much money you have and how much you spend.

Make copies of the following worksheets and use them to create your spending plan. Complete a new worksheet every time your situation changes.

ACTIVITY

Monthly Income

STEP 1: Identify Income – Estimate your monthly income. If your income varies, keep track of it for several months. Then, determine your average monthly income by dividing the total income by the number of months. You may need to estimate what your income will be if you cut back on the hours you work or aren't able to work at all, due to your medical condition.

SOURCES	PER MONTH
After-Tax Wages	$ _____
Tips or Bonuses	$ _____
Child Support	$ _____
Alimony/Maintenance Payment	$ _____
Unemployment Compensation	$ _____
Social Security or Supplemental Security Income	$ _____
Public Assistance	$ _____
Food Stamps	$ _____
Tax Refunds	$ _____
Interest/Dividends	$ _____
Other	$ _____
Total Income:	$ _____

Monthly Income (continued)

STEP 2: List Expenses – Estimate your monthly expenses. You may need to antici-pate more money for medical expenses to manage your fibromyalgia. If you aren't sure how much you spend for such things as meals, gas or entertainment, start a spending notebook. Record what you spend on everything for the next two or three months. At the end of that time, add what you have spent, divide the sum by the number of months, and use the results to complete the worksheet.

SOURCES	PER MONTH
Rent or Mortgage	$ _____
Heat, Electricity and Water	$ _____
Telephone	$ _____
Groceries	$ _____
Medications (include prescription drugs, nutritional supplements	$ _____
and over-the-counter medications)	$ _____
Transportation (bus fare, car payment, gas, repairs, etc.)	$ _____
Insurance (car, health, life, disability, homeowners, etc.)	$ _____
Clothing/Uniforms	$ _____
Doctor/Dentist Bills (include increased expenses due to fibromyalgia)	$ _____
Pet Care	$ _____
Loan/Credit Card Payments	$ _____
Entertainment (movies, eating out, etc.)	$ _____
Miscellaneous (classes, gifts, vacations, union dues, etc.)	$ _____
Taxes	$ _____
Savings*	$ _____
Other	$ _____
Total Expenses:	$ _____

*If you think of saving money as a regular monthly expense, you will be more likely to stick to a savings plan.

STEP 3: Compare Income and Expenses	
Write down your total monthly income (from Step 1)	$ _____
Write down your total monthly expenses (from Step 2)	$ _____
Subtract expenses from income and list amount here	$ _____

STEP 4: Set Priorities and Make Changes – Do you have money remaining at the end of the month? Congratulations! If you take advantage of this surplus (by putting it into an investment or a savings account, for example), you will be even further ahead. If you came up short, don't be discouraged. Take another look at your spending plan to find places where you may be able to increase your income, cut expenses or both. Use this space to summarize your financial inventory.

1. I completed the "Assets, Liabilities and Net Worth" worksheet on _____ (date).

2. I made copies of the "Spending Plan" worksheet and completed the first one on _____ (date).

3. My ideas for increasing my income, reducing my expenses or both include:

Choosing an Insurance Plan

Having good medical coverage may be the most important asset people with fibromyalgia have. Whether you have an individual or group policy, you should acquaint yourself with what your plan offers and find out how you can add to it or make certain changes to it. Use the following checklist to evaluate your policy.

❏ YES ❏ NO

Does it cover fibromyalgia? Read the fine print. Find out if the policy has a clause that excludes coverage of fibromyalgia or related conditions.

❏ YES ❏ NO

Does it offer outpatient and inpatient care? Look for a policy that offers coverage for doctor's visits and other outpatient services as well as coverage for surgery and hospital stays.

❏ YES ❏ NO

Can you choose your doctor? If you have a managed care policy, such as those offered by a Preferred Provider Organization (PPO) or a Health Maintenance Organization (HMO), you may be limited to the health-care providers in their network. If your doctor is not in the network, you may have to find a new doctor.

❏ YES ❏ NO

Does the plan include rehabilitation coverage? Rehabilitation coverage

includes physical, occupational and vocational therapy. Also look for coverage of assistive devices.

❏ YES ❏ NO

Are prescription drugs covered? Ask to see the insurance plan's "formulary," or list of drugs the plan covers. Make sure the medications you are currently taking are covered.

❏ YES ❏ NO

Are laboratory and other monitoring procedures covered? These procedures should be covered not only for diagnosing conditions, but also for monitoring your response to medications and therapies.

❏ YES ❏ NO

What are the costs? Be sure to weigh the benefits of the policy against the costs (such as the premium, deductible, copayment, out-of-pocket cap and any annual or lifetime maximum benefits).

❏ YES ❏ NO

Have you checked out the plan's report card? Check to see if a consumer group has rated the health-care plan for customer satisfaction and quality of life.

❏ YES ❏ NO

How's their service? Test the plan's customer service. Call the insurer's customer service number and see how quickly you get help.

Look For Alternative Therapy Coverage

If you rely on alternative therapies to manage your fibromyalgia symptoms, then you should check to see if those therapies are covered by your insurance. More and more, insurance companies are including complementary therapies, such as counseling or chiropractic care, in the health coverage.

If alternative treatments are not covered as a standard benefit, ask your plan administrator about covering them as a rider to your plan. Riders provide additional coverage for services not usually covered in a standard benefits package. Riders may cost an additional $5 to $30 per month and may cover — with a co-payment — such treatments as acupuncture or massage.

Another option is the flexible spending account, which is offered by many employers. Participants commit a certain amount of each paycheck — before taxes — into an account for medical expenses that are not covered by other insurance.

Talk to your plan administrator or contact your insurance company to see how you can get coverage for your alternative therapies. Here are some therapies to look for in your policy:

- Physical therapy
- Psychological counseling
- Acupuncture
- Pain clinic coverage

- Chiropractic care
- Massage therapy
- Well-being and lifestyle classes

Take Charge

The Arthritis Foundation and the National Endowment for Financial Education (NEFE) offer a booklet called *Take Charge: Money Matters and Your Arthritis*. *Take Charge* can help you develop a financial plan. To order, call 800/283-7800 or visit www.arthritis.org.

GOOD LIVING
GOOD LIVING
GOOD LIVING
GOOD LIVING
GOOD LIVING
GOOD LIVING
GOOD LIVING
GOOD LIVING
GOOD LIVING
GOOD LIVING

RESOURCES

The mission of the Arthritis Foundation is to improve lives through leadership in the prevention, control and cure of arthritis and related diseases.

As a nonprofit organization, the Arthritis Foundation relies on your contributions to fund research, programs and services. You can make a difference in people's lives by becoming a member of the Arthritis Foundation. Please contact your local chapter or call 800/933-0032. You will receive materials about the benefits of Arthritis Foundation membership, including the award-winning bimonthly magazine Arthritis Today. Log on to the Foundation Web site, www.arthritis.org, for more information about arthritis, Arthritis Foundation resources or to find the chapter nearest you.

Programs and Services

Physician referral – Most Arthritis Foundation chapters can provide a list of doctors in your area who specialize in the evaluation and treatment of arthritis and arthritis-related diseases.

Exercise programs – The Arthritis Foundation sponsors, develops and coordinates exercise programs for people with arthritis, featuring specially trained instructors. These programs include:

- Walk With Ease – This course, accompanied by a book, shows you ways to develop a walking routine for fitness.

- *PACE** (People with Arthritis Can Exercise) – These courses feature gentle movements to increase joint flexibility, range of motion, stamina and muscle strength. An accompanying video is available for home use.

- Arthritis Foundation Aquatic Program – These water exercise programs help relieve strain on muscles and joints. An accompanying PEP (Pool Exercise Program) video is available for home use.

Educational and Support Groups – The Arthritis Foundation sponsors mutual-support groups that provide opportunities for discussion and problem-solving among people with arthritis. In addition, the Arthritis Foundation offers courses designed to help people actively manage their particular disease through exercise, medications, relaxation techniques, pain management, nutrition and more. These classes include the Arthritis Self-Help Course and the Fibromyalgia Self-Help Course.

Information and Products

Find the latest information about arthritis, including research, medications, government advocacy, programs and services, through one of the many information resources offered by the Arthritis Foundation:

www.arthritis.org

Information about arthritis is available 24 hours a day on the Internet at the Arthritis Foundation's interactive, comprehensive Web site. Find news about arthritis, ways to get involved, and a variety of useful arthritis products, including books, brochures, videos and more.

Arthritis Answers

Call toll-free at 800/283-7800 for 24-hour, automated information about arthritis and Arthritis Foundation resources. Trained volunteers and staff also are available at your local Arthritis Foundation chapter to answer questions or refer you to physicians and other resources. For general questions about arthritis, you also can call 404/872-7100, Ext. 1, or email questions to help@arthritis.org.

Publications

The Arthritis Foundation offers many publications to educate people with arthritis, as well as their families and friends, about diagnosis, medications, exercise, diet, pain management and more.

- Books – The Arthritis Foundation publishes a variety of books on arthritis to help you understand and manage your condition, live a healthier life, and cope with the emotional challenges that come with a chronic illness. Order books directly at www.arthritis.org, or by calling 800/207-8633. All Arthritis Foundation books are available in retail bookstores.

- Brochures – The Arthritis Foundation offers brochures containing concise, understandable information on the many arthritis-related diseases and conditions. Topics include surgery, the latest medications, guidance for working with your doctors, and self-managing your illness. Single copies are available free of charge at www.arthritis.org, or by calling 800/283-7800.

- *Arthritis Today* – This award-winning, bimonthly magazine provides interesting feature articles in each issue, providing the latest information on research, new treatments, trends and tips from experts and readers to help you manage arthritis. *Arthritis Today* also publishes a bonus seventh issue in the fall. This issue is the annual Buyer's Guide, which serves as a one-stop resource for products and services that make life with arthritis and related diseases easier and more enjoyable. The listings directory is also available online at www.arthritis.org. A one-year subscription to *Arthritis Today* is included as a benefit when you become a member of the Arthritis Foundation. Annual membership is $20 and helps fund research to find cures for arthritis. Call 800/933-0032 for information.

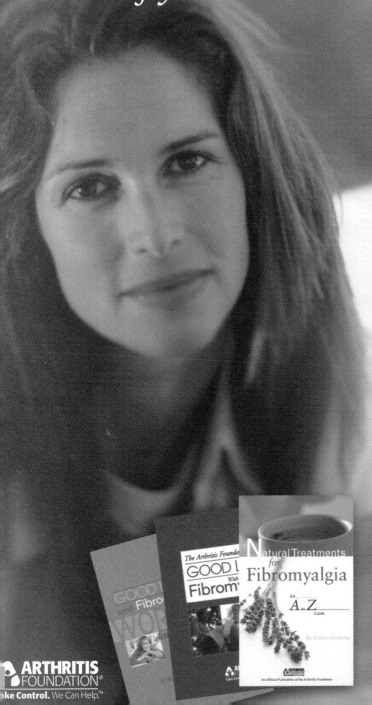

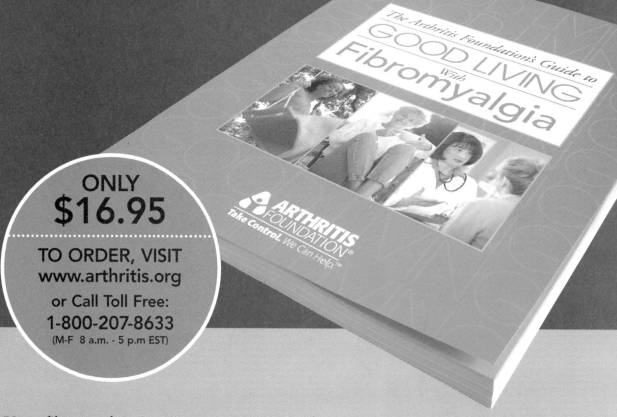
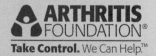